Special Diets:
Tightwad Tara's Guide

For Kile

ISBN 978-1-257-82448-9

Forward

"*Everyone should have access to healthy food, and Tara has found a way to help anyone enjoy wholesome and allergen-free alternatives. I have experienced, with my step-son, the challenges of implementing a special diet and understand how time consuming and expensive it can become. No matter what your food budget is, learning Tara's tips for meal planning, bulk shopping and cooking techniques, can save valuable time and amplify the enjoyment of cooking. Tara's vast knowledge of ingredients and nutrition is perfectly complemented by her organizational talents and her experience in special diets.*"

John H. Hicks, MD

Table of Contents

INTRODUCTION

CHAPTER 1 *Getting Started on a Special Diet*

CHAPTER 2 *Planning When to cook*

CHAPTER 3 *Planning What to Cook*

CHAPTER 4 *Planning How to Cook*

Introduction

NEWS OF A SPECIAL DIET

People use special diets for many reasons. Some people use diet to control their weight, alleviate health concerns, or even to maintain a healthy lifestyle. On a quest to heal our middle child from his hyperactivity and behavior problems, I began to research diet to control his erratic behavior. Just weeks before his fourth birthday, we received the devastating news that he was diagnosed autistic and ADHD and that he would likely never be able to talk or maintain a normal life. Our psychiatric doctors were skeptical that diet would alleviate our son's behavior problems and autistic symptoms and discouraged diet to manage his behavior. My husband and I felt strongly that diet can control behavior and agreed to try modifying his diet to see if it would help him. We already ate food free of additives, preservatives, artificial flavorings and colors. We decided to also implement the GFCF (gluten-free/casein free) diet, which is commonly used for autistic children.

First we eliminated dairy and casein and then we eliminated gluten. Within weeks, his hyperactivity was under control and he began to speak. Over time on the special diet, his uncontrolled darting stopped, his focus increased, he began sleeping through night, his arm flapping stopped, mood swings were under control, and behavior continued to improve. If he ate gluten or casein, the undesirable behaviors would return.

The diet did help tremendously with his behavior problems and autistic symptoms, but there was something beyond just gluten and casein. Even with intense supplemental treatment, his damaged intestines were having difficulty healing. After about two years, he became sensitive to even more foods. He continued to improve cognitively, his speech was increasing steadily, and he began making friends but began having difficulty controlling his anger, frustration and self-mutilation (biting himself) when he was upset.

The anger episodes lasted about nine months until we went on vacation in the summer, and his anger outbursts and many autistic symptoms disappeared. The symptoms reappeared at the end of our vacation, which led me to believe that something he was eating was again creating problems. We researched the Feingold Diet and realized that most of the food he was eating was causing him to bite himself. We realized his body was having trouble processing phenols and salicylates. Next we eliminated foods high in salicylates, which includes foods such as apples, oranges, red grapes, almonds, cucumbers, and green peppers. Although these foods are extremely healthy, his body was unable to process them at the time. After we eliminated the salicylates, his angry outbursts, lack of self control, and self-biting stopped and his bowel movements were normal for the first time since early infancy. His mood was steady and he was happy. After the removal of the salicylates, we noticed certain foods were still causing behavior reactions. Foods containing benzoates such as peas, cauliflower, spinach, and broccoli were also causing behavior problems similar to the foods containing salicylates. We then discovered a majority of foods with sulfur such as eggs, artificial amino acids, or soy could also not be processed and caused a reaction similar to the reaction of gluten and casein. Fortunately we were able to use digestive enzymes to correct the problem of his inability to process salicylates and phenols and he can consume them without problems. The gluten and casein continue to be a problem and many of his autistic symptoms will come back if he consumes either one.

Although eliminating these foods from his diet did not completely heal his body, it did alleviate behavior and comprehension problems while the body continued to heal. With a combination of food, supplements, fermented foods, and diet control, we have been able to continue to reverse his autism and heal his body. Someday he'll be able to reintroduce the foods he once loved.

THE JOURNEY TO SAVING TIME AND MONEY

The journey for saving money began after the birth of our first child. Prior to having children, my husband and I decided that we would both work full time. But shortly after our first child was born, we both felt one parent should stay home. It was then that we decided to raise our children on a single income.

In the spring of 2000, I quit my job to focus on raising our children. Money was tight but our marriage was strong, and we were able to focus on forming strong relationships with our children. Each week we would pay the bills and cringe. Although our family unit was strong, we had a difficult time financially. I pondered ways to make extra money from home. I considered a home sales business or even working part time but these options didn't fit with the dynamics of our family.

IT'S NOT WHAT YOU MAKE, IT'S WHAT YOU SAVE

It was after the birth of our second son that I realized it wasn't how much money we made, but how much money we saved. We were about $600 short each month to pay our bills. We began to look for options to reduce our bills. First we refinanced our home, which saved $175 a month. We sold our newer vehicle for an older model, which lowered our car payments $250 a month. Our children already wore previously owned clothes, which saved hundreds of dollars each year, and we chose to participate in preschool activities locally that were free or very low cost. We rented movies and music from the library and spent our days playing at the park or joining in playgroups with other children. We used cloth diapers and homemade diaper wipes. We were saving money but not quite enough.

Originally, it was my quest to eat healthy that helped decrease our grocery bills. I began cooking from scratch in order to affordably incorporate organic and natural foods into our diet and eliminate food additives.

I found that cooking from scratch increased my time in the kitchen very little, and we were able to cut our grocery bills nearly in half. By our third year of marriage, we had reduced our grocery budget from $80 a week to $40 a week, saving us $160 a month. Not only was our grocery budget decreased, but we also were able to eat mostly organic, without food additives and preservatives. We were able to save enough money each month so that I didn't have to work.

THE JOURNEY TO SAVING TIME

The journey to saving time began after the birth of our second son. He was born a beautiful, healthy baby boy. He progressed normally in all areas of his life and even walked and talked earlier than other children his age. I was pregnant with our third child shortly after his first birthday. By the time he reached 18 months old, he began to lose his speech. His behavior became extremely hyperactive and he could never be left unattended. The only time he would settle down was if he were watching TV and even then it would only last a short time. At this point in time I had a difficult 4-year-old, a hyperactive 2-year-old and a newborn baby. This proved to be a challenge for me while I tried to cook dinner each day. I began to use different methods to try to reduce my time in the kitchen in order to focus on my family.

We came to realize our second son's behavior challenges were brought about by a number of food intolerances — food intolerances that we were able to manage by using several special diets. We were easily able to incorporate the special diets through the time- and money-saving techniques we were already using on our regular diet.

Although our middle son has recovered from many of his behavior challenges, we still use these cooking methods in our busy life. There are times now when I work full time and my husband works overtime or travels. Our children are busy in activities and we live a very active life.

Common Questions About Special Diets

WHAT IS A FOOD ALLERGY OR FOOD INTOLERANCE?

The difference between food allergy and food intolerance is that an allergy is an immune response to a food that the body sees as harmful, and an intolerance is an adverse reaction that does not involve the immune system. An anaphylactic reaction is a severe allergic reaction that is rapid onset and may cause death. People are on special diets for many different reasons. Many people choose diet to control emotions, behavior or weight loss and others are forced into special diets by severe intolerance or allergy to foods.

DO SPECIAL DIETS WORK?

For many people, special diets are the key to controlling their health. What foods you choose to fuel your body will determine how well a diet works. I have found that a diet typically fails when a person fails to follow the diet. Often being too lax with a special diet will sabotage all efforts. I also have found people will do well for a few weeks or even a few months but lack perseverance to maintain the special diet in order to allow healing.

WHAT IF THE SPECIAL DIET DOESN'T WORK?

Don't give up. The special diet may need to be further examined. In extreme cases, the special diet may extend beyond food itself. For example, someone with a gluten intolerance may react to anything containing gluten including vinegar, vanilla, shampoo, conditioner, soaps, toothpaste, glue, products containing sticky adhesive such as tape, stickers, bandages or Band-Aids, play dough, glue, papier-mâché, clays, envelopes, and certain school supplies, cleaners, and medications.

Also consider whether this is the correct diet to be on. For example, if the GFCF diet doesn't work for an autistic or ADHD child, try the SCD diet. Maybe the Feingold Diet would be a better fit. Maybe there are more severe intolerances involved that are not showing up on medical or blood tests. Neither wheat nor diary show up on an IGG blood test as being severe to our son, yet we know that both of these substances will cause a severe adverse reaction.

HOW STRICT SHOULD I BE ON AN ALLERGY-FREE OR SPECIAL DIET?

That depends on your doctor and the health condition being dealt with. People doing special diets treating conditions such as cancer, allergies, celiac disease, Crohn's disease, autism, or other autoimmune disorder should be strict. Be sure to talk to a specialist (nutritionist, dietitian, doctor, etc.) about the seriousness of the allergy, intolerance, or sensitivity. Get a second opinion if necessary. I was told by our pediatrician and also by top doctors from a well-known hospital in our state that a special diet was not necessary for our son and to not even try a special diet. I tried it anyway. Within two weeks of being on the special diet, his hyperactivity stopped, he began to sleep through the night, and he quit darting and having emotional mood swings.

I CAN'T AFFORD AN ALLERGY-FREE OR SPECIAL DIET!

It is true that many allergy-free or health foods are more expensive than many conventional foods, especially if using convenience foods. I have found that by creating my own mixes, sauces, baked goods, and breads and eliminating most convenient foods that I significantly reduce the cost of allergy free groceries. I also find that being organized and having a meal plan will also greatly reduce my grocery bill. In 2009 my average weekly grocery bill for my family of five was $75. I spent over $80 a week in 1999, when my husband and I ate primarily convenience foods, and I spent the same amount of time cooking in the kitchen. When I began cooking from scratch in 2001, our grocery bills dropped from $80 a week to $40 a week — for my husband, myself, and two small children. Changing habits is one of the most important factors in lowering grocery bills.

BUT DOESN'T THAT TAKE TOO MUCH TIME?

Not really. Changing cooking habits will greatly reduce time in the kitchen. I cook about 2 ½ hours a week (not including lunch assembly time). This will be discussed in the cooking methods section. I cook almost everything from scratch and we eat primarily organic food.

MY FAMILY HATES THE ALLERGY-FREE AND SPECIAL FOOD!

Focus on what you CAN have not on what you can't have. Keep experimenting. Find a cookbook or cookbooks that have reliable recipes. I have found the recipes for gluten-free cooking are nearly always reliable in all of Bette Hagman's books including The Gluten Free Gourmet Cooks Fast and Healthy. I also find recipes from Martha Stewart are almost always reliable. Although they may not be allergy-free, the recipes can easily be converted to what you need and are easy to make. Also remember to keep it simple when cooking allergy-free. A meal of a simple meat and steamed vegetables is quick and easy. Just because it is allergy-free doesn't mean that it has to be unflavorful.

ARE ALLERGY-FREE OR SPECIAL DIETS HEALTHY?

With any diet, it is your choice of food that makes the diet healthy. Just because it is allergy-free doesn't mean it is beneficial to your body. What food you choose to put into your body will make a difference as to how well and how fast your body will heal. A diet rich in fruits, vegetables, and high quality meat — low in sugar and high in fiber — will give the body the energy it needs to heal, as opposed to soft drinks, candy, snack crackers, fast food, french fries, chicken nuggets, and chips.

IS THIS SPECIAL DIET FOREVER?

The amount of time you need to be on a special diet depends on your medical condition and the advice of your nutritionist or other diet specialist. Some diets last months, some last years, and others are a lifetime change. If you are also working to heal the body along with a special diet, the special diet often does not have to be followed once the body has healed.

Saving Time and Money on a Special Diet

Chapter 1

GETTING STARTED

Often I am approached by people who want to change their diet but feel that they don't have time to dedicate to eating healthy and fear that a special diet will cost too much to implement. Having a plan is the key to saving time and money on a special diet.

Time and money can both be saved by planning when to cook, what to cook, and how to cook each meal. Meals can be prepared at a time when it is most convenient to you. Knowing what you will cook each day will alleviate the last-minute stress of deciding what to eat for dinner, and using different methods to cook will save money and time in preparation. Money can be saved by learning to preserve food by freezing, dehydrating, canning and even fermenting. Money can also be saved by having a grocery budget and using a time budget will help you manage your time. In this book you will learn how to:

- **Plan when to cook**

- **Plan what to cook**

- **Plan how to cook**

- **Preserve food**

- **Budget time and money**

Chapter 2

PLANNING WHEN TO COOK

Having a schedule and knowing the best time to cook will help reduce cooking times in the kitchen and help organize meals.

SCHEDULE TIME TO COOK

Having a schedule to your day is important because it helps determine when you will cook dinner and eat. If your day is unscheduled, you may have a hard time finding time to cook and often you will be rushed when you do cook. Most children thrive on a routine and schedule, especially special needs children. This helps create security with your family, especially if you have young children. Consider scheduling meals and snack times to eliminate constant snacking throughout the day. If scheduled properly, cooking meals can take significantly less time.

A schedule doesn't have to be specific and can work around general times in the day.

A sample schedule on a non-workday is as follows:

7 a.m.	Breakfast
8 a.m.	Take kids to school
8:30-11:30 a.m.	Playtime, get groceries, run errands
Noon	Lunch
1-2:45 p.m.	Nap for kids, cook supper, clean house, phone calls, exercise, personal time
3:15 p.m.	Pick kids up from school
3:45-4:45 p.m.	Talk with family
5 p.m.	Set kitchen table and be sure dinner is warming
5:30 p.m.	Eat

6:45-8:20 p.m.	Family time
8:30-9 p.m.	Read books and get ready for bed
9 p.m.	Bedtime. After children are in bed, pack lunches for the next day; set out clothes, coats, bags; do laundry and enjoy free time. Cook dinner if necessary for the following day.

A sample schedule for a workday is as follows:

7 a.m.	Breakfast
7:30 a.m.	Leave for work
5 p.m.	Home from work
5-5:30 p.m.	Talk with family
5:30 p.m.	Set kitchen table and be sure dinner is warming
6 p.m.	Eat
7-8:20 p.m.	Family Time
8:30-9 p.m.	Read books and get ready for bed
9 p.m.	Bedtime. After children are in bed, pack lunches for the next day; set out clothes, coats, bags; do laundry and enjoy free time. Cook dinner if necessary for the following day.

In this schedule, dinner isn't necessarily cooked on a workday. The meal can be prepared prior to that day such as the day before, the evening before, the weekend before or even sometimes cooked a month ahead of time. Also notice that on a non-workday, cooking is done at 1 pm not at 5 pm. This eliminates distraction, decreases cooking time and the rush to get dinner on the table therefore reducing stress.

CHOOSE THE BEST TIME TO COOK

Cooking can be done at many different times during the day. What time works best for you depends on your schedule. Cooking at 5 pm may be a stressful time to get dinner ready. Preparing dinner earlier in the day may eliminate distractions. Cooking with children in the mornings, during the winter or even in the evenings after supper may work better in your schedule. If you are working full time, schedule a low maintenance meal for that evening. Prepare the meal earlier in the week then refrigerate or freeze it or have the ingredients prepared and ready to throw together when it is time for dinner. The weekends can be an ideal time to prepare meals. The following methods may give you ideas as to when may be a good time to cook or when cooking may fit into your schedule. Each family is different and not every time will work for every family.

The following are six time formats that can be used to cook:

Time 1 – Immediate Cooking

Cook immediately before you eat each day. This is one of the most common times to cook, but it also may be the most inefficient and most difficult. Time is wasted by cooking a single meal every day. Often people begin to feel hungry then rush to the pantry to see what can be thrown together for dinner. This type of poor planning will also cost more money than planning out the meals. This method may work best for your family, but if it doesn't, look at the following methods to see if these fit better into your schedule.

Time 2 – Cook or Prepare Earlier or Later in the Day

Almost any recipe or meal can be prepared in advance. Cooking can be done earlier or later in the day, such as nap time, prior to everyone waking, later in the evening or even after everyone goes to bed. Meals can also be prepared in the morning and placed in a Crock-Pot to cook all day.

See the Planning How to Cook section to get ideas on what can be done at this time. Prepare foods such as cutting raw vegetables, make grilled cheese sandwiches that can be put in refrigerator until supper, put food into a Crock-Pot, get pans out for later use, brown meat and put in fridge, or anything that may save time before the meal. By getting the meal organized and at least semi-ready, the 5 p.m. rush to get dinner on the table can be eliminated.

Time 3 – Cook Only One or Two Days a Week
Cooking only once or twice a week can save time and energy. Meals can be coordinated to use similar ingredients in order to reduce time (see Piggy-Back Cooking). Several batches of the same meal can be cooked then frozen or three to four days' worth of meals can be prepared at the same time to eliminate cooking and cleaning on the following days. Those meals can either be refrigerated or frozen depending on what is prepared and how quickly it will be eaten. This method saves time in preparing the meal and also in washing dishes.

Time 4 – Bulk Cooking
Cooking bulk items includes making a large quantity of a recipe or making several batches of a meal or recipe. Try to cook bulk items in the mornings or after supper in the evenings. Items such as pasta sauce, taco sauce, pancakes to freeze, soups to freeze, main dishes to freeze, or other items that do not pertain to an immediate meal can be prepared during family time, after supper, during the day or during any free time. This is a great time to include children during cooking. Children learn valuable cooking skills and have fun making their own food. Even a 2-year-old can pour ingredients into a mixer and help stir. Cooking together is a wonderful way to spend time as a family.

Time 5 – Cook Once a Month
Another option is cooking once a month then freezing the meals. There are several books on the market that explain how to do this and even give menu plans and grocery lists. At this time, I do not believe there is a once-a-month cooking book for special diets so you would have to create your own plan. This method would save the most time and money. To do this method, plan out meals for one month, get the groceries for those meals and then spend one day cooking the meals that will then

go into the freezer. The key to making this work is planning meals that coordinate with one another (see Piggy-Back Cooking) and a large freezer for storing.

Time 6 – Start a Cooking Club

Start a cooking club with people on the same special diet. Meet one time per month in which each person brings 10 of the same meals to a meeting to share. The meals are then lined up and each person takes home 10 meals that their family would like to put in their freezer. Some people assemble the meal at the meeting and some people bring the meal already assembled. The advantage to a cooking club is the time saved in cooking and money can be saved if you choose a cost-effective recipe to share. The disadvantage is that you have no control over what is added to each dish. Some families are stricter than others on the ingredients in each prepared dish. This method may work if you lived in a large city or had a group of people on the same diet such as a gluten-free diet commonly used for celiac disease.

Chapter 3

PLANNING WHAT TO COOK

Knowing what you will have for dinner in advance is another way to save time and money. If you know what you will eat, then you will be able to coordinate meals and ingredients to eliminate food waste and also avoid rushing to get dinner on the table at the end of the day.

To get started, keep a list of favorite meals nearby and label what cookbooks to find them in. Next, make a meal plan each week. Plan one to two weeks of meals at a time and write them down and place in a visible spot.

KEEP A RECIPE NOTEBOOK

It may be difficult to think of four, two, or even one week's worth of meals at one time. To gain ideas as what to cook, go through cookbooks and favorite recipes and make a master list in a notebook of all the meals that your family would like to eat. While writing down the recipe name, also note the page number and cookbook that it came from for quick reference. This will take some time to compile but will save time and effort in the long run. Keep the master list in a notebook that's easy to access then when you need an idea for a meal. Redo the list every year or two or when your family's needs change. It may be too overwhelming to do the list all at once. Try doing a cookbook a day or a week. Find time while riding in the car, a break at work, after the kids go to bed, while the family watches a movie, or any free time.

The following chart is an example of how recipes can be recorded into a notebook. Include the cookbook title, write down the recipe and page number and then write a special note about the recipe, if needed, indicating special ingredients or family favorites. The cookbooks used for this example are a local Mothers of Preschoolers cookbook, Better Homes and Gardens, and Old Threshers local cookbook.

If you are just starting a special diet, this is a great way to find recipes that you already have or can be easily adjusted that will fit well into your diet.

Our Favorite Recipes- Master List

MOPS Cookbook
Breakfast Casserole pg. 68
Chicken Tetrazzini pg. 79 .... takes long time to make this
Chicken Roll-ups pg. 86 .... Family loves these
Easy Chicken and Rice pg. 90

Better Homes and Gardens Cookbook
Scrambled Egg Pizza pg. 268 .... make a cheese sauce also
Farmer Casserole pg. 272 .... Family loves this
Sloppy Joes pg. 363
Spinach Pasta Noodles pg. 380
Chicken Fiesta Salad pg. 456

Old Threshers Cookbook
Sour Dough Starter pg. 24
Crock Pot Pizza pg. 46
Gluten-Free Brownies pg. 114 .... quick recipe
Pasta Sauce pg. 187 .... use tomato paste, 2 cans
Strawberry Sherbet pg. 193
Zucchini Jam pg. 184 .... good use for garden zucchini

MAKE A MENU PLAN

After you have a master meal list, write down what you are going to have
for dinner each night and post it where you can see it or in a planner
so you don't forget what you bought groceries for. Keep a daily planner
that has a meal planning section for each day of the year. Write the meal
planned for the day on each day for one, two or more weeks. Be sure
to include the page number and cookbook that the recipe is found in
to save time in searching for the recipe. Easier recipes that are cooked
often may not require a cookbook if the recipe is memorized. Next, write
down the ingredients that are needed for each meal in the planner. Also
include a running grocery list that can be added to during the week as
something runs out.

Monday	Tuesday	Wednesday	Thursday	Friday	Saturday	Sunday
Taco soup	beans & rice	crock pot chicken	Chicken tacos	pizza	chicken pot pie	omelets and hash browns
recipe card	pg. 95 Peace L.	Crock Pot pamphlet	pg. 195 Old T	DD Pg. 96	pg. 164 Peace L.	

Grocery List:

kidney beans, 1 bag

tortilla shells

cheese, 2 cheddar, 1 mozzarella

frozen veggies, 1 mixed, 1 broccoli

butter alternative

green peppers, celery, lettuce, carrots

deli meat, 1 lb.

deli cheese, 1 lb.

eggs, 2 dozen

milk, 2 gal.

juice

tomato sauce

The 4 Week Plan

Recently I began to plan dinners four weeks at a time, and I immediately trimmed over $50 off of my total grocery bill for a four-week time period ($600 per year). To save money, I also do not go to the grocery store more than once a week. On the four-week cycle, I get all my dried goods, cereals, shredded cheese to freeze, chips, frozen items, cooking staples and other items I will need over the next four weeks on the first week. On weeks two through four, I only get fruit, vegetables, dairy products and perishables. On the first week I spend about $100. On weeks two through four, I spend about $65 each week. This enables me to keep my groceries under $300 a month at the grocery store. I also purchase food in bulk from a health food co-op and organic chickens from a local farmer. Over the course of a year, this totals about $400, or a $30 a month average, to be added onto my total grocery bill.

Flexibility

Be flexible with your meal schedule. Meal plans can often change with busy family schedules. If a meal needs to be changed, switch a meal that will take less time to prepare with a meal that is more labor intensive. Keep prepared meals in your freezer for emergencies.

Look for simple recipes or a mix of simple recipes with a few complex recipes when meal planning. Some meals take much more time than others to prepare. During a week try to plan several simple meals along with one or two that will take a little bit more time. When cooking the meals that take more time, try to cook two or three days' worth of meals at one time that way you only have to cook two or three times in one week.

In order to save money, look for varied price per meals. Some meals are cheaper than others. Try to have meals average 75 cents or less per person with a total grocery bill of $75 per week or less. Organic chicken is expensive but if you have bean burritos the same week, the price per meal is averaged out. An organic chicken meal may cost over $1 per person but a bean burrito meal can cost as little as 35 cents per person. You could also make a note of the recipe cost next to the recipe the first time you make it. It may seem like a lot of work at first, but you will get a true estimate of how much you are spending on each recipe. This may be a way for you to lower your grocery bills.

Chapter 4

PLANNING HOW TO COOK

There are many different methods of cooking that may be used in order to complete a meal. Not every method will be applicable to everyone and some methods may work better than others, depending on family dynamics and schedule. Most people begin pulling out ingredients at 5 pm to cook supper. The following methods will help eliminate the five o'clock rush to get dinner on the table and place the cooking at a more convenient time.

The method you use for cooking will greatly be determined by your lifestyle and preference for cooking. Each of these methods may not work for every person. One method may work better for a person who does not work outside of the home, and a different method may work better for a person working full time. A person with small children will use methods differently than a person keeping up with a teenager's schedule or even more different than a person cooking with no children at all. These are a few methods that can be used for efficient meal planning.

Method 1 – Bulk Prepared Mixes

Bulk prepared mixes are made by taking the dry ingredients from favorite recipes and placing them in a large container. Keep bulk prepared mixes in the pantry for quick cooking. To make the bulk prepared mix, make the recipe five to 10 times the size of the original recipe. Label the container with a slip of paper and place on top of the mix with the cookbook and page number as to where the recipe is located. Another way to label the container is to make a copy of the recipe and tape the recipe directly to the container. Also make any notes in the cookbook or directly on the recipe taped to the container for any changes that need to be made. Mixes that can be used include: pancake mix, gluten-free flour mixes, cream of mushroom soup mix, spaghetti sauce mix, sausage seasoning mix, ranch dressing spices, and Italian dressing spices. Spice mixes can be made about one time per year. Soup mixes can be made about two times per year and the other mixes can be made about every four months or so. Keep the mixes in a cool dry place such as a refrigerator or freezer to extend the longevity of the mixes.

The following is an example of how to take a recipe and make it into a bulk prepared mix.

Classic Pancakes — Original Recipe

¾	cup gluten-free flour mix
2	teaspoons baking powder
½	teaspoon xanthan gum
½	teaspoon salt
1	teaspoon sugar
2	eggs, well beaten
½	cup milk alternative
2	tablespoons oil

Beat together eggs, milk, and oil. Sift together flour, baking powder, salt, xanthan gum, and sugar in another bowl. Stir into egg mixture until all ingredients are well blended. Cook on hot griddle. Be sure to spread the batter to make it thin on the griddle or the middle may not get cooked evenly.

To make this into a prepared mix, first sort the dry and wet ingredients. Next, increase the amounts of each ingredient in only the dry ingredients list. This recipe is 6 times the amount of the original. Measure out and store the dry ingredients until ready to use.

Calculate the math on the dry ingredients:

Classic Pancakes — Bulk Prepared Mix Recipe

> ¾ cup gluten-free flour mix x 6 = 4 ½ cups
>
> 2 teaspoons baking powder x 6 = 12 tsp (or 4 Tbsp)
>
> ½ teaspoon xanthan gum x 6 = 3 teaspoons
>
> ½ teaspoon salt x 6 = 3 teaspoons
>
> 1 teaspoon sugar x 6 = 6 teaspoons (or 2 Tbsp)
>
> 2 eggs, well beaten (do not calculate)
>
> ½ cup milk alternative (do not calculate)
>
> 2 tablespoons oil (do not calculate)

Do not calculate the wet ingredients because they will not be added until later.

Here is the revised version for the prepared mix method:

Classic Pancakes

In a large container add:

> 4 ½ cups gluten-free flour mix
>
> 4 tablespoons baking powder
>
> 3 teaspoons xanthan gum
>
> 3 teaspoons salt
>
> 2 tablespoons sugar

Next calculate the total amount of dry ingredients that was used in the original recipe:

¾ cup flour + 2 teaspoons baking powder + ½ teaspoon xanthan gum + ½ teaspoon salt + 1 teaspoon sugar = total dry ingredients.

Add the teaspoons: 2 teaspoons baking powder + ½ teaspoon xanthan gum + ½ teaspoon salt + 1 teaspoon sugar = 4 teaspoons dry ingredients. Then add the flour. The total amount of dry ingredients used will be ¾ cup + 4 teaspoons.

We arrived at this number because the original recipe called for ¾ cup flour and the total of the other dried goods equals 4 teaspoons (2 teaspoons + ½ teaspoon + ½ teaspoon +1 teaspoon = 4 teaspoons) so the total amount of dry ingredients used will be ¾ cup + 4 teaspoons.

When ready to make pancakes, measure out ¾ cup plus 4 teaspoons of dry mix into a bowl. Then add:

2 eggs, well beaten

½ cup milk alternative

2 tablespoons oil

Beat together eggs, milk, and oil. Add this mixture to the dry mix that has been measured out and stir until all ingredients are well blended. Cook on hot griddle. Be sure to spread the batter to make it thin on the griddle or the middle may not get cooked evenly.

By taking the dry ingredients of a recipe and storing them in a large quantity, time will be saved in mixing and also in washing dishes. Be sure to clearly label each container as to what mix is inside.

Method 2 – Assembly Line

When my kids were young — before I was preparing allergy-free/ intolerance-free meals — I would order organic flour 50 pounds at a time, simply to save money and time. I then would line up large plastic sealable bags (25 or 30) and fill each with 3 ½ cups of flour. Then I added 2 teaspoons of salt to each bag. Then 2 tablespoons sugar and 2 tablespoons powdered milk. This is the equivalent to a purchased bread mix in a box at the store, except much cheaper. Organic bread mixes can cost as much as $5 or $6. This organic bread mix prepared at home costs 32 cents. By doing an assembly line, time is saved washing dishes and in preparing food and money is saved buying the food in bulk. Time is saved because the ingredients are only taken out one time, dishes are only washed once and when it is time to cook, most of the preparation has already been done. When it is time to cook the bread, simply pour out the mix and add a few wet ingredients. This can be done with many items. Try this with pizza mixes, cake mixes, bread mixes, pancake mixes, and pie crust mixes. This method can be used for any recipes that would be used frequently or could be purchased in the store in a box. This method can be used in combination with the in-a-jar cooking method. It is best to do this method without distractions so you do not lose count when you are trying to assemble your mixes.

The following is an example of how we use the Gluten-Free Bread Mix for the Machine recipe in the assembly-line method.

Gluten-Free Bread for Machine — Original Recipe

> 3 ⅛ cups gluten-free flour mix
>
> 1 ½ teaspoons salt
>
> 3 ½ teaspoons xanthan gum
>
> 2 tablespoons brown sugar or blackstrap molasses
>
> ¼ teaspoon ascorbic acid (opt.)
>
> 3 eggs, beaten
>
> 1 ⅛ cup warm water
>
> 3 tablespoons oil
>
> 2 ¼ teaspoons yeast or 1 pkg. of yeast

Place ingredients in bread machine according to manufacturer's directions. Press start button. Or, dissolve yeast in warm water for 5 min. Combine flour, salt, xanthan gum, and brown sugar in a small bowl. Combine eggs, water with dissolved yeast, and oil in bread machine bucket. Add dry ingredients. Set to "light" cycle. Press start.

Gluten Free Bread for Machine — Assembly-Line Recipe

Combine the following dry ingredients in a sealed container or plastic bag that seals. There are approximately 2 cups of flour per pound so 25 pounds of flour will give you approximately 16 batches or enough flour for 16 loaves of bread. Add the specified amount to each container or bag and store in a cool dry place until ready to use.

> 3 ⅛ cups gluten-free flour mix
>
> 1 ½ teaspoons salt
>
> 3 ½ teaspoons xanthan gum
>
> 2 tablespoons brown sugar
>
> ¼ teaspoon ascorbic acid (opt.)

When ready to make bread, using the ingredients below, combine the water and yeast first and let sit three to five minutes. Next, combine the eggs and oil together and add to the water and yeast mixture.

> 3 eggs, beaten
> 1 ⅛ cup warm water
> 3 tablespoons oil
> 1¼ teaspoons yeast or 1 pkg.

Place ingredients in bread machine according to manufacturer's directions. Either add the liquids first, then the dry mix stored in the bag or add the dry mix first, then the liquids. Press start button.

The ingredients didn't change in the new recipe, just the time as to when each ingredient is mixed up into the recipe. A gluten-free bread mix will cost $5 to $6 in the store not including the wet ingredients. This mix costs around $2.50 to make including the wet ingredients.

Method 3 – In-a-Jar

In-a-Jar and Assembly-Line methods are very similar. The difference between them is the quantity made. In-a-Jar method has a smaller quantity of mixes, usually less than five, and the Assembly-Line has a large quantity of mixes created.

Prepare cookies, cakes, brownies, breads, or whatever mix you would buy in a box at the store by putting the dry ingredients in a jar with a lid then later adding the wet ingredients. This type of cooking mix is popular around the holiday seasons and is known as "Gifts-in-a-Jar." Go through your recipe to determine the dry ingredients. Add them to a jar. Label the jar as to what is in it and either put what needs to be added also on the label or indicate where the recipe is located so that you may add the wet ingredients later. A piece of paper can be slipped on top of the mix that gives the page number of the recipe, what the recipe is, and any other notes. Masking tape could also be added to the jar with the same information. Simply use the mix when you are ready. Look up the recipe according to your label. Add the wet ingredients and then follow the rest of the recipe. This makes for quick cooking and is great for toddlers or kids with ADHD because of the short mixing time. Try this for any of your favorite recipes. The jars also make great decorations and gifts. This method works well when you need food quickly.

The following is an example of how to change a recipe for an in-a-jar method. This is the original recipe adapted from Bob's Red Mill Vanilla Almond Sugar Cookies.

Almond Coconut Sugar Cookies

> 2 c. sugar
> 1 c. coconut oil, butter or margarine
> ⅔ c. almond milk or other milk alternative
> 4 t. vanilla (optional)
> 1 ½ c. rice flour
> ⅔ c. coconut flour
> 4 T. potato or tapioca starch
> 1 t. baking powder
> 1 t. baking soda
> 1 c. almonds, sliced (optional)

Cream together the coconut oil and sugar. Add vanilla and almond milk. In a separate bowl, combine rice flour, coconut flour, tapioca starch, baking powder and baking soda. Add dry ingredients to wet ingredients and mix until just blended. Roll into 1" balls and flatten slightly on a greased cookie sheet. Bake 10-12 minutes at 350 degrees. Remove from the pan gently while still warm. Let the cookies cool.

Use quart or pint jars to hold the recipe ingredients. In order to use pint jars, the recipe must be converted to a smaller recipe. The pint jars hold less than 1 ½ cup of dry mix so the above recipe will have to be divided in two. In order to use quart jars, the recipe could be left as is. To use pint jars, first cut the recipe in half. Next add the dry ingredients to the jar then place the jar in a dry place until ready to use. Third, add the wet ingredients when ready to make the recipe.

To use pint jars, calculate the math:
Almond Coconut Sugar Cookies (for pint size jars)

  2 cups sugar ÷ 2 = 1 cup sugar

  1 ½ cups rice flour ÷ 2 = 3/4 cup rice flour

  ⅔ c. coconut flour ÷ 2 = 1/3 cup coconut flour

  4 tablespoons potato or tapioca starch ÷ 2 = 4 tablespoons
  potato or tapioca starch

  1 teaspoons baking powder ÷ 2 = ½ teaspoons baking powder

  1 teaspoon baking soda ÷ 2 = ½ teaspoon baking soda

  1 cup coconut oil, butter or margarine ÷ 2 = ½ cup coconut oil,
  butter or margarine

  ⅔ cup almond milk or other milk alternative ÷ 2 = 1/3 cup
  almond milk or other milk alternative

  4 teaspoons vanilla (optional) ÷ 2 = 2 teaspoons vanilla
  (optional)

  1 cup almonds, sliced ÷ 2 = ½ almonds, sliced

The following is the smaller, revised version of the recipe:
Almond Coconut Sugar Cookies In-a-Jar

In a pint jar, combine the following:

  1 c. sugar

  ¾ c. rice flour

  ⅓ c. coconut flour

  2 T. potato or tapioca starch

  ½ t. baking powder

  ½ t. baking soda

Place jar in dark, dry area until ready to use.

Ingredients to add:

  ½ c. coconut oil, butter or margarine

  ⅓ c. almond milk or other milk alternative

  2 t. vanilla (optional)

  ½ c. almonds, sliced (optional)

In a bowl, beat coconut oil, butter or margarine until light and fluffy.

Add vanilla. Alternately add pint jar mix and milk or milk alternative and blend just until combined. Add sliced almonds if desired. Do not over mix. Roll into 1" balls and flatten slightly on a greased cookie sheet. Bake 10-12 minutes at 350 degrees. Remove from the pan gently while still warm. Let the cookies cool.

Again, the ingredients didn't change for the recipe, just the time that it is mixed up. Be sure to label the jar with the recipe and also the page number and cookbook it came from. Also remember if you reduce a recipe, also reduce the pan size. Make four to six jars at a time to save time in cleaning and mixing later. If you bake four to five cakes per year this means that you would only have to mix up this recipe one time per year. This recipe works best for cakes and cookies, but it will work for other recipes such as bread, soup, or dip mixes. By using this method, time can be saved by mixing several batches at once and also by having less dishes to wash. Money can be saved by combining your own mix.

Method 4 – Batch and Freeze

Many recipes can be made in a large quantity and then frozen. Some meals work better than others. When making a meal or side dish, make two or four. It won't take much more time but will save time in cooking and cleaning later because the ingredients need to be taken out only once and the dishes for preparation also need to be washed only once. This method can be used with burritos, pasta sauce, egg rolls, Spanish rice, applesauce, spaghetti sauce, taco sauce, refried beans, jams, enchilada sauce, pancakes, French toast, cookies, cakes, cupcakes, pie crusts, main dishes, pesto, jellies, and many others. This method would also work well with once-a-month cooking or cooking only a few days a week.

The following is an example of how to increase a recipe for a Batch-and-Freeze method. This is the original recipe. If this recipe is quadrupled, it will be enough for 5 meals or the pancakes can be warmed individually in the toaster as needed. A typical family of four can make this recipe four to five times per year. Recipes can be increased by any number. Increase the recipe only by the amount you can eat before the food storage life in the freezer expires.

Classic Gluten-Free Pancakes — Original Recipe

2	eggs, well beaten
½	cup milk alternative
2	tablespoons oil
¾	cup gluten-free flour mix
2	teaspoons baking powder
½	teaspoon xanthan gum
½	teaspoon salt
1	teaspoon sugar

Beat together eggs, milk and oil. Sift together flour, baking powder, salt, xanthan gum, and sugar in another bowl. Stir into egg mixture until all ingredients are well blended. Cook on hot griddle. Be sure to spread the batter to make it thin on the griddle or the middle may not get cooked evenly.

Now increase the recipe by 4 for each ingredient. Follow the directions to make the pancakes.

Classic Gluten-Free Pancakes — Batch-and-Freeze Recipe

2	eggs, well beaten x 4 = 8 eggs
½	cup milk alternative x 4 = 2 cups
2	tablespoons oil x 4 = 8 tablespoons
¾	cup gluten-free flour mix x 4 = 3 cups
2	teaspoons baking powder x 4 = 8 teaspoons
½	teaspoon xanthan gum x 4 = 2 teaspoons
½	teaspoon salt x 4 = 2 teaspoons
1	teaspoon sugar x 4 = 4 teaspoons

Here is the revised version for the Batch-and-Freeze method:

Classic Gluten-Free Pancakes

8	eggs, well beaten
2	cups milk alternative
8	tablespoons oil
3	cups gluten-free flour mix
8	teaspoons baking powder
2	teaspoons xanthan gum
2	teaspoons salt
4	teaspoons sugar

Beat together eggs, milk and oil. Sift together flour, baking powder, salt, xanthan gum, and sugar in another bowl. Stir into egg mixture until all ingredients are well blended. Cook on hot griddle. Be sure to spread the batter to make it thin on the griddle or the middle may not get cooked evenly.

Once the recipe is complete, freeze the pancakes in a freezer safe container until ready to use. The pancakes can be thawed out in the refrigerator, cooked in a toaster or toaster oven, or warmed in the oven or microwave when ready to use.

Method 5 – Prepare Individual Ingredients and Freeze

Individual ingredients can be prepared at a convenient time then used later in cooking in order to save time. For example, try cooking meats such as ground beef, 5 pounds at a time. Ground beef will freeze for up to 3 months. Freeze the meat in 1-pound packages and simply pull the meat from the freezer when you are ready to assemble the meal. This will eliminate cooking and cleaning time. Often the meat will not even need to be thawed out before using. For ingredients such as chicken broth, sort 2 cups at a time or in ice cube trays then freeze the containers or trays. This is also a good way to save money if items can be found on sale. Individual ingredients that freeze well include: cooked bacon, bread slices, bread crumbs, meatballs, fresh fruit, fresh vegetables, flours that will not be used quickly, nuts, shredded zucchini, block cheese that has been shredded, and many other ingredients. Sauces and purees can also be frozen in ice cube trays then transferred to another container. Leftover sauce from an open can also freezes well. Experiment with many foods.

The Cheese Freeze

I once found a sale on organic block cheese, $1 for 8 oz. I purchased $50 worth of cheese then shredded the cheese in my food processor at home. Next I froze the shredded cheese. At the time of purchase, non-organic cheese was $1.75 an 8 oz. block and organic cheese was $5 for an 8 oz. block. I saved $37.50 total if comparing the organic cheese on sale with non-organic cheese and a savings of $200 if comparing the organic cheese on sale with other organic cheese. Either way, it was worth my time and money to freeze the ingredients.

Method 6 – Piggy-Back Cooking

Piggy-Back Cooking is a method using similar ingredients on consecutive days in order to reduce the cost of groceries, eliminate excess food or unusable leftovers, and save time in cooking. Plan your meals to coordinate ingredients with the meal for the next day. This saves time and money. One week may go like this:

MONDAY – Spaghetti Pie (Brown extra hamburger for Tuesday)

TUESDAY – Tacos (Use browned meat from Monday, chop extra raw veggies for Thursday and Saturday)

WEDNESDAY – Whole chicken in a Crock-Pot and Steamed Veggies (Make stock from the chicken)

THURSDAY – Chicken Salad Wraps (Use chicken from Wednesday and raw veggies from Tuesday)

FRIDAY – Pizza (May use extra chopped veggies from Tuesday)

SATURDAY – Chicken soup (Use veggies from Tuesday and chicken and chicken stock from Wednesday)

SUNDAY – Sandwiches

This week of meals will take about an hour or so of cooking. Tuesday and Thursday will have no cooking; just meal preparation that can be done earlier in the day. Pizza takes only 10 minutes total and the chicken will take only one to two minutes to prepare and 15 minutes or so to take it off the bone. On Saturday it is again just assembly and let it warm on the stove. Make stock from the cooked chicken leftovers and freeze it or use it in other recipes during the week. Also use the extra chicken in meals for the week or freeze the extra chicken for later use.

Here is another example of meal piggy-back for a week:
MONDAY – Hamburgers on the Grill and Greek Salad. Use 2 pounds of hamburger. Make 1 pound into hamburger patties, and fry 1 pound into taco meat to be used on Tuesday. The Greek salad has tomatoes, cucumbers and green peppers. Chop extra tomatoes for Tuesday and slice extra cucumbers and green peppers for Wednesday.

TUESDAY – Tacos, using taco meat cooked on Monday. Also use tomatoes from Monday. Serve with salsa and chips. If the salsa is homemade, thaw it from the freezer or use canned salsa. If tomatoes are in season, you could make fresh salsa on Monday while you are preparing the other vegetables. This would also allow time for flavors to blend.

WEDNESDAY – BLTs, using bacon from the freezer that has been pre-baked and frozen using Method 4 of freezing individual ingredients for later use. It will take 15 seconds in the microwave to cook the bacon. Use the vegetables pre-cut from Monday. Slice fresh tomatoes to use. Slice extra tomatoes and clean extra lettuce for Thursday.

THURSDAY – Submarine Sandwich. French bread could be homemade or purchased. Homemade bread will save money, but purchased bread may save time. Two loaves of French bread could be made for about 32 cents. One loaf at the store will cost about $1.50. This is a savings of $2.36. Freeze the extra slices of bread to be toasted later with spaghetti or other pasta dish. If making homemade bread, pre-mix the dry ingredients for the pizza crust on Friday.

FRIDAY – Pizza. Use pre-mixed crust from Thursday and tomatoes cut on Thursday. Thaw out sauce from freezer, make it from scratch or use sauce from a jar. Cheese can be fresh or from the freezer.

SATURDAY – Grilled Chicken and Lettuce Salad. Cook extra chicken for Sunday.

SUNDAY – Chicken salad sandwiches using chicken from Saturday.

During this example week Monday will be a longer cooking day. Tuesday and Wednesday will be low maintenance cooking days if the salsa is pre-made or purchased. Thursday can be a quick cooking day if the bread is purchased or it can also be a longer cooking day. Friday will take less than 10 minutes. Saturday the time will be spent in front of the grill and Sunday will only be assembly from Saturday's leftovers.

Method 7 – Adapt-a-Recipe
Many recipes can be adapted to fit dietary needs. With a little practice and experimenting, it will be easier to recognize a potential recipe that will fit specific dietary needs. When looking for a recipe, look for what ingredients do work in the recipe. Also look for what can be easily substituted. If a recipe calls for wheat flour, cheese, milk, and is topped with peanuts, don't try to adapt the recipe if the person has wheat, milk and peanut allergies and intolerances. But if a recipe has all acceptable ingredients except for the type of flour, try to make a substitution. The following is an example of adaptable recipes.

The following is a recipe for classic pancakes.

Classic Pancakes

> ¾ cup flour
> 2 teaspoons baking powder
> ½ teaspoon salt
> 1 teaspoon sugar
> 2 eggs, well beaten
> ½ cup milk
> 2 tablespoons oil

Beat together eggs, milk and oil. Sift together flour, baking powder, salt, and sugar in another bowl. Stir into egg mixture until all ingredients are well blended. Cook on hot griddle.

Make substitutions to the original recipe. Look to see what works. A person allergic to gluten and dairy can have baking powder, salt, sugar, eggs and oil. A person who is intolerant to wheat flour can first make the substitution of the flours. Typically xanthan gum is used in baking with gluten-free flours. The conversion is usually 1 teaspoon of xanthan gum for every 1 cup of gluten-free flour so add xanthan gum to this recipe. A person who is also intolerant to milk can substitute a milk alternative to the recipe. If the new recipe was spread out in the center with a spoon to make a thinner pancake, then the middle would cook evenly with the rest of the pancake. Alter the directions to reflect the new pancakes. The following recipe is the altered version of the original recipe.

Classic Pancakes — Adapted Recipe

¾	cup gluten-free flour mix
½	teaspoon xanthan gum
2	teaspoons baking powder
½	teaspoon salt
1	teaspoon sugar
2	eggs, well beaten
½	cup milk alternative
2	tablespoons oil

Beat together eggs, milk and oil. Sift together flour, baking powder, salt, xanthan gum and sugar in another bowl. Stir into egg mixture until all ingredients are well blended. Cook on hot griddle. Be sure to spread the batter to make it thin on the griddle or the middle may not get cooked evenly.

This recipe has been easily adapted to be gluten- and dairy-free. The method of cooking is the same for this recipe and the ingredients are only slightly changed.

Chapter 5

PRESERVATION OF FOOD

Preservation of food is an excellent way to not only eat healthy but also save money on your grocery bill. The advantage to preserving food is that you have control of the ingredients that are in or around your foods. It is also a wonderful way to spend time as a family, either gardening or preparing produce for preservation.

One way to save money is to grow your own produce. Another way to save money is to purchase produce while it is in season, at a reduced price, and then preserve it through freezing, canning, fermenting, or drying so it can be used throughout the year. This may also save time because the preparation of the food is done once, therefore saving time in cleaning kitchen utensils and preparing the produce at a convenient time. For example, we grow our own tomatoes. When the tomatoes are ready to be harvested in late summer, we then freeze the tomato halves to be used in place of canned whole tomatoes for soups throughout the year. We also can the tomato juice, can salsa, or eat the tomatoes fresh.

As a general rule of thumb, if you can purchase an item in a can or frozen at the grocery store, you can probably can or freeze the same item or something similar at home. If you are unsure if an item can be frozen, consider if the item can be purchased frozen at the grocery store. Food companies will use the most efficient and best food preparation methods in order to maximize profits for grocery items.

FREEZING

Freezing can be used to preserve fruits, vegetables, meats, and precooked foods. It is an excellent way to retain the color and fresh flavor of foods. It is also the fastest, least time-consuming method for preserving.

Food can still spoil if using the freezer method. To prevent spoilage, start with fresh, high-quality food, freeze the food below 0° Fahrenheit, and use sanitary conditions in preparing the food to freeze.

When preparing fruit for canning or freezing, the fruit can be packed in fruit juice for a healthier option, as opposed to adding white sugar to the mixture. Water can also be used. When making jams and jellies, a special fruit pectin can be purchased in which sugar is not needed and fruit juice can be used as a replacement. This no-sugar pectin can be purchased at a local discount store, grocery store, or wherever canning supplies are sold. Avoid artificial sweeteners.

Packaging for freezing should be free of moisture, odorless, tasteless, grease-proof, and able to be tightly closed. The best types of packaging include:

Glass canning and freezing jars are easy to clean and can be reused. Plastic screw-tight lids can be used to seal the containers.

Plastic freezer containers can be stored easily in the freezer. They are not as fragile as glass freezer jars and can be used for versatile storage other than freezing.

Flexible plastic freezer bags can be used for many items. Be sure they are labeled for freezer use. Do not heat the freezer bags.

Vacuum packaging is an excellent way to keep food three to five times longer than regular storage life. They will also eliminate odors — like those of onions or green peppers — that can ruin the taste of other foods if stored with other methods. Freezer vacuum bags can be boiled, microwaved, and reused.

Freezing Tips:
Be sure items to be frozen are wrapped properly prior to freezing. This will prevent freezer burn. Meat should be kept in its original packaging. Freeze the food as quickly as possible so that it will not form large ice crystals between the fibers of the food, which can physically change the

food while in storage.

To reheat frozen foods, cook main dishes and pies in the oven. Cooking time will be longer if the food is frozen. To decrease cooking time, thaw the food in the refrigerator before placing in the oven.

To reheat soups, heat the food to serving temperature on the stove.

Foods such as sandwiches, cakes, cookies, and fruits can be served after thawing.

Foods such as cookies, candy, and fruit can be served while still frozen.

To thaw food from the freezer, place the food in the refrigerator overnight. Food can also be placed in cold water to thaw or in a microwave on the defrost cycle. Remember that a microwave will kill all nutrients in the food.

Food should not be refrozen unless in an emergency. Foods thawed partially that still contain ice crystals can be refrozen but you may lose the color, flavor or texture of the food. If a food has been thawed slowly to a temperature of 40°, the food may be unsafe to refreeze.

Freeze sandwiches

An advantage to freezing sandwiches is that it may save time and money to "mass freeze" in an assembly line method. This is particularly helpful for packing lunches.

To freeze sandwiches, use day-old bread, spread with butter or butter alternative, and then add fillings. The best fillings to use include cheese, chicken, meat, peanut butter, nut butters, fish, and egg yolk mixtures. Wrap the sandwich in freezer film and freeze on a tray. When the sandwiches are frozen, transfer them to a large freezer bag or freezer safe container. Be sure to label the sandwiches.

DEHYDRATING

It's easy to dry foods, and dried foods are convenient to store. Many foods can be dried including fruits, vegetables, and meat. Fruits and vegetables can be eaten plain or added to main dishes, jams, and other cooked foods. They can also be rehydrated and used like fresh foods.

There are several different methods of dehydration. The most reliable method is to use an electric dehydrator. Food can be dried in less than 24 hours, resulting in food that has been dried evenly and quickly. Before purchasing this appliance, consider the price of the dehydrator and how much you will use it to be sure this method will be cost-effective. Other methods that can be used include natural drying and oven drying. Natural drying, such as by the sun, can be used when the temperature is over 90 degrees and there is low humidity and low pollution. The oven can also be used for small quantities, but the operating costs of using an oven could be high compared to using a food dryer.

CANNING

Canning is an easy, low-cost way to preserve fresh foods. Although it is a relatively easy process, it does take some time and special attention. Canning is an excellent way to preserve fresh foods, sauces, jams, and other items for a long period of time.

Canning involves packing recipes or fresh food in a special glass jar, sealing the jar with special lids, then heating the jars in a boiling water bath to seal the lid to limit the possibility of food spoilage. If you plan to can, the "Ball Blue Book" of preserving is an excellent source for recipes and procedures in all aspects of preserving, including canning, freezing, and dehydrating.

FERMENTING

Fermented foods are made by allowing foods to set at room temperature (around 72 degrees) until the food is fermented. Vegetables stored in a brine need to set three to seven days. Whole grains, beans, lentils, raw nuts and seeds, and whole-grain flours need to ferment at least seven hours. During this time, friendly bacteria reproduce and convert sugars and starches into lactic acid. The fermentation process is slowed by placing the food into the refrigerator. Although refrigeration does not stop the fermentation process, it does slow it down. Foods that are made from natural fermentation include sourdough breads, fermented pickles, sauerkraut, kefir, yogurt, sour cream, sour cream butter, and cultured vegetables. Although friendly bacteria does not need to be added to most fermented foods, a culture can be purchased for making these foods to ensure the friendly bacteria grows well. Fermented foods are believed to aid in digestion and are often tolerated well by people with digestion or intestinal problems.

Chapter 6

MAKING A BUDGET FOR TIME AND MONEY

Budget Your Time

People are often familiar with making a budget for money, but also make a budget for your time. Make a chart or list of how your time is spent on a daily basis. Keep track of what you do each hour and journal where it goes. The key to saving time is to step back and observe how your time is spent then re-evaluate how to better spend your time.

Go through your schedule and determine when you have free time. For some people it may be only on the weekends. Others have a break time at work. Riding in the car, train or bus also counts for free time. Look for the small spaces of time such as waiting in line or waiting to pick up children. Using the small spaces of time to do work may leave larger spaces of time later on. If you feel that you have absolutely no free time, determine where your time is spent. Where are you spending most of your time? Do you work too many hours? Are you constantly running to your children's activities? How much TV do you watch? How many hours are you on the Internet each day? Do you spend too much time on e-mail, texting or Facebook? How often are you on the phone? Go through your schedule and determine what is most important. Determine what can be eliminated or shortened from your schedule. Set a timer for yourself while you are cleaning or reading a magazine. Set a time limit for your phone conversations, Internet and e-mail if necessary. If you are talking on the phone, clean at the same time. Take your lunch to work instead of going out to eat. Learn to number your days. Time is spent but is never given back. A wise person knows time is a commodity. Each person is given 24 hours each day. How we spend that time depends on us. How you spend your time will be your top priority in your life. How you spend your time reflects what is most important to you.

Don't Waste Time

People often ask me where I find the time to cook everything from scratch, have it organic and cook for food allergies and intolerances all at the same time. My response is good planning. I often carry a pen and planner with me to take notes or write reminders to myself. I do not waste time. I plan when I will cook and what I will cook during my spare moments that are often short. I plan during my breaks at work, during car rides, while waiting for my kids at activities or school, in a doctor's office, at the playground, or even while watching a TV show with my children. Notice when you have time or when you aren't doing anything. This may be a good time to plan your cooking. I spend approximately ½ hour every four weeks planning what meals we will have and making my grocery list. I spend about 10 minutes each week reviewing my meal plan and making a grocery list.

MAKING A GROCERY BUDGET

The first step in making a grocery budget is finding out how much you are currently spending on groceries. Keep four weeks of grocery receipts and receipts from eating out. Write out each item purchased, along with its cost. Next, see where your money is being spent, then evaluate what can be reduced or switched in grocery purchases. Write out your basic needs and then make the budget. Try changing recipes and varying menu choices to have a more economically balanced diet. The following is an example of making a grocery budget:

Write out groceries purchased in one month

Fruit and Veggies	Meat
Monthly total $72	Monthly deli meat $24
Weekly average $18	Monthly other meat $18
	Total monthly meat $42
	Weekly average meat $10.50

Baked Goods (tortillas, bread, etc.)

Dairy

Monthly total $20	Monthly total milk $30
Weekly average $5	Monthly total shredded cheese $20
	Monthly total chunk cheese $20
	Monthly deli sliced cheese $20
	Monthly total yogurt $20
	Monthly total ice-cream $14
	Monthly total other dairy $8
	Total monthly dairy $132
	Weekly average dairy $33

Baking Supplies

Chips and snacks

Monthly total $60

Monthly chips $20

Weekly average $15

Monthly crackers $10

Monthly dried fruit $24

Monthly cookies $8

Monthly snack total $62

Weekly snack average $15.50

Miscellaneous

Monthly average juice $12

Monthly average cereal $60

Monthly average organic eggs $14

Monthly canned tomatoes or tomato products $30

Monthly other groceries $20

Total monthly miscellaneous $136

Total weekly miscellaneous $34

Next, calculate total weekly average spending:

Fruit and Veggies	$18.00
Meat	$10.50
Baked Goods	$ 5.00
Dairy	$33.00
Baking Supplies	$15.00
Chips and Snacks	$15.50
Miscellaneous	$34.00
Total weekly groceries	**$131.00**

Third, find where groceries can be reduced. In this example, spending seems to be fine on fruit and vegetables, meat, and baked goods. However, when we look at dairy, $60 a month is being spent on cheese. Cheese should be reduced significantly. The block cheese could be completely eliminated or reduced to $2 to $5 a month. This would save $15 a month or $3.75 a week. The shredded cheese could be purchased on sale at $1.25 a package instead of $2.00 and then frozen until needed. This would save $7.50 in a month or $1.88 in a week. Powdered milk could be purchased for baking and cooking instead of liquid milk. This would save about $4 a month. Yogurt could be made homemade thus making the total yogurt expense $6 a month instead of $20. This would save $14 a month or $3.50 a week. Ice cream could be eliminated or reduced to $3 a month which would save $11 a month and $2.75 a week. Baking supplies will stay the same. Chips and crackers could be reduced by consuming less with a savings of $5 a month each. Dried fruit could be reduced by $14 a month or $3.50 a week by not consuming as much. This money would be better spent on fresh fruit. Cookies could be eliminated or reduced to $2.50 a month with a savings of $5.50 a month or $1.38 a week. Cereal could be purchased on sale with a savings of $10 a month and eggs could be purchased at a local farm with a savings of $5 a month. Tomatoes could be homegrown and canned or made into sauce or salsa in the late summer. This would reduce the monthly tomato cost about to $5 a month or less.

Other groceries may be reduced by purchasing items in bulk or on sale. This budget could further be reduced if all items were purchased on sale. Milk may be $1 cheaper per gallon at one store and vegetables may be over $5 overall cheaper at the same store. This would save an additional $8 a week by shopping two different stores.

Fourth, rewrite the budget:

Groceries Weekly Average

Fruits and veggies	$13.00
Meat	$10.50
Baked goods	$ 5.00

Dairy

Milk	$ 4.75
Shredded cheese	$ 3.12
Deli cheese	$ 4.00
Chunk cheese	$ 1.25
Yogurt	$ 1.50
Ice cream	$ .75
Other	$ 2.00

Baking supplies	$15.00

Chips and snacks

Chips	$ 3.75
Crackers	$ 1.25
Dried fruit	$ 2.50
Cookies	$ .50

Miscellaneous

Juice	$ 3.00
Cereal	$ 8.50
Eggs	$ 2.25
Canned tomatoes	$ 1.25
Other	$17.00
Total groceries	**$97.75**

In this example, we were able to easily reduce groceries $28.75 per week and $115.00 per month by changing a few bad snacking habits, making a few things from scratch and purchasing items on sale. This budget could even be further decreased by making more items from scratch, purchasing more items on sale and preserving food from a home grown garden.

Holy Cow

Recently we purchased   of a cow. The cow costs $2.50 per pound and we had the meat cut to our specifications. The cow was farm-raised and grass-fed with no antibiotics or hormones given to the cow. Hamburger is currently $2.99 per pound at our local grocery store and steak is much higher. By purchasing meat in bulk we were able to have very high quality meat and save $0.50 or more per pound.

TIPS TO SAVING MONEY IN GROCERY SHOPPING

In order to save money in cooking:

- Know where to shop

- Know the price value of each item

- Know what is best quality

- Be aware of deceptive advertising, claims for lowest pricing, coupons, etc.

- Be willing to change habits

Other ways of saving money on the grocery budget are knowing where to purchase each item, accurate cost comparisons, and determining the time and cost of making items at home.

KNOW WHERE TO SHOP

The price paid for each item will depend greatly on your location, grocery store, and access to discount health food. High prices do not reflect high quality nor does a low price indicate the best deal. The grocery budget is the easiest place to save money because it can be flexible. Local health food stores may have items that are typically higher priced than other local grocery stores, but they also carry many hard to find baking and food items for specialty diets. Wait for items such bread mixes and cold cereal to go on sale then purchase a six-month supply. If Envirokids cereal is $5 a box at the health food store, $4 a box at the grocery store and $2.50 a box on sale through a health food co-op, then eating three boxes per week would cost $780, $624, and $390 respectively per year. A savings of $390 per year on cold cereal can be made by simply knowing where to purchase products at a lesser price.

If this same pricing strategy was used on all purchased food, literally thousands of dollars could be saved each year on groceries.

KNOW PRICE VALUE

Calculate the price per ounce or pound of foods when comparing costs of similar items. Foods are sold in different size containers and by calculating the cost of items made, you will be able to determine if it is cost effective to purchase that item or to make it yourself.

Although the price difference per ounce of a particular item may seem like a small amount, calculate the cost of the item to get a better gauge as to how much is being spent. For example, a small loaf of homemade gluten-free bread uses approximately 3 cups of flour or 24 oz. per loaf. If a bean blend is used to make bread, it will cost approximately $2.62 for the flour mix (flour, plus salt, baking powder and xanthan gum). If approximately 55 loaves of bread are made per year, it will cost about $141.10 for dried goods to make homemade bread by pre-mixing the flour at home and a pre-mixed bread package from the store will cost about $4.50 per loaf or about $247.50 per year. About $106.40 per year could be saved by pre-mixing flour mixes. If a store-bought loaf cost approximately $5.50 per loaf or $302.50 per year, almost $161.40 per year or almost $13.50 per month could be saved by making bread from scratch.

KNOW WHAT IS BEST QUALITY

Sometimes higher quality products appear to be more expensive. Be sure to buy high quality brands because often generic brands contain bleached flour or sugar, dyed brown sugar, or unwanted added ingredients. Even the brand of flour used in baking can affect the size of a bread loaf or brownie size.

BE AWARE OF DECEPTIVE ADVERTISING, CLAIMS FOR LOWEST PRICING, COUPONS, ETC.

I have found that grocery stores that claim to have "Lowest Prices, Always" or "Save Money Like Never Before" have several items that are lower priced than most stores but overall do not have the lowest prices. These stores will reduce the price on items such as milk, eggs or other high-demand item to get people to come into a retail store hoping they will make additional purchases in the store. I also found that when I stopped shopping at these mega-discount grocery stores my grocery bills were reduced by over $20 a week or $80 a month.

Coupons are often used to reduce the price of an item. Coupons are often used on new products or even higher priced items. A coupon can save you money if it is an item that you were planning to buy. Sometimes the cost of the brand the coupon is being used for will actually cost higher than a similar product, therefore, costing more money to use the coupon. Be sure to calculate the math on the coupon savings verses a similar product or making the product at home. Often, coupons do not save the most amount of money. Organized shopping and making products from scratch save more money overall.

BE WILLING TO CHANGE HABITS

Changing grocery stores, items purchased at the store or even the type of meal prepared can be difficult. Don't try to change everything at once, work on one habit at a time. Decide what would be the best or easiest habit to start with. Plan how you will change the habit and continue the "new normal" for at least thirty days. Repeat changing habits until you have reached the "new normal" in all areas.

STORE BOUGHT VS. HOMEMADE

Before starting an allergy-free/intolerance-free diet, I would have said it is almost always cheaper to cook something homemade as opposed to purchasing it at the store. In fact, Amy Dacyczyn, author of the Tightwad Gazette, says that the only thing that is cheaper store bought than homemade is macaroni and cheese and I have also found that to be true. However, with cooking on a special diet, it is sometimes cheaper to purchase products in the store in a pre-made mix or pre-made product rather than making them homemade. The best way to figure the cost comparison is to do a cost analysis of the recipe. The price of a product can be calculated per ounce, cup or ½ cup for easier conversion and comparison. In order to calculate the cost of a product, take the amount in the package and divide it by the price of the product. Prices will fluctuate for each product depending on where you live, the price of fuel, supply and demand and other factors.

The following in an example of how to calculate price per package:
Bob's Red Mill Gluten-Free Baking Flour Mix purchased from the grocery store is 22 oz. and approximately $3.44 per package. Divide the price of the package ($3.44) by the number of ounces (22) and the price per ounce is 16 cents.

In observing the gluten-free flour mixes, the following are the approximate cost per ounce for each flour mix:

Dark Bean Flour with garbanzo bean flour	10.5 cents
Dark Bean Flour with Garfava bean flour	11.6 cents
Beans and Rice Mix	11.10 cents
Light Bean Flour	12 cents
Featherlight Mix	12.16 cents
Pre-Mix Bob's Red Mill GF Flour mix	16 cents
Bette Hagman mix from the Internet shipping)	28 cents (plus

The cost difference does not seem like much, but look at usage. In a typical bread, cake or cookie recipe, approximately 3 cups or 24 oz. of gluten-free flour is used. Look at these prices again:

Dark Bean Flour with garbanzo bean flour	$2.52
Beans and Rice Mix	$2.66
Dark Bean Flour with Garfava bean flour	$2.78

Light Bean Flour	$2.88
Featherlight Mix	$2.92
Pre-Mix Bob's Red Mill Flour mix	$3.84
Bette Hagman mix from the Internet	$6.79 (plus shipping)

It costs approximately $1.32 more per loaf of bread, cake or batch of cookies for a pre-mixed flour mix as opposed to mixing it on your own compared to Bob's Red Mill pre-mixed flour and $4.27 more per loaf if using Bette Hagman's pre-mixed flour purchased on the Internet. I make one loaf of bread every week and it would save me nearly $69 per year to make my own flour mix as opposed to purchasing pre-mixed flour from Bob's Red Mill and over $222.04 per year to make my own flour mix as opposed to purchasing Bette Hagman's pre-mixed flour from the internet.

Better Bread

Sometimes it is cheaper to buy a mix. I found Bob's Red Mill Gluten-Free Bread Mix on sale through a health food co-op at 30 percent off. In a cost analysis of bread we can see what is most cost-effective. This particular purchased bread mix will make approximately   more bread than my bread machine mix from scratch.

My bread homemade	$2.66
Bread Mix	$4.50
Bread Mix on sale	$2.98
Premade Loaf of bread at the store	$4.50-$6.25

It is more cost-effective to make bread form scratch unless the mix is on sale. Although the bread mix on sale is slightly higher priced than my homemade bread, the loaf is actually larger than my loaf and can be made a little faster. When the bread mix goes on sale, purchase a three-to four-month supply. In this case it saves time and money to purchase a mix from the store.

Be sure product comparison is for similar products. For regular wheat bread, one person may purchase a loaf for 50 cents at Wal-Mart and another person may purchase a similar loaf for 35 cents at Aldi. A homemade loaf can be made for less than 35 cents but the homemade loaf is all organic, and contains no additives or preservatives. To find a loaf of bread at the store similar to the homemade loaf, the cost would be around $4 per loaf; therefore, homemade bread is not only more healthy but also cheaper.

When choosing to make food from scratch or purchasing it pre-made from the store, consider the time, money and effort involved. Making food from a mix doesn't always save time and often will cost considerably more. However, if a mix saves time and money it would be more time-efficient and cost-effective to purchase the mix. Also consider the ingredients in the purchased mix. Most pre-packaged mixes contain undesirable ingredients. However, specialty food mixes tend to contain ingredients that are more natural as opposed to chemically altered pre-made food. In conclusion, calculate what a recipe will cost to make and compare the time to make it with the amount of money needed to make the recipe. If the mix is cheaper and the ingredients are healthy, buy the mix. If not, make the mix yourself.

In conclusion, both time and money can both be saved by having a plan of when to cook, what to cook, how to cook and budgeting. How much money saved on groceries can also be determined by how detailed a cost comparison is done on comparable groceries. Most people will compare only what can be purchased at the store. Factor in what can be made at home without considering the time consumed making the certain product when doing an initial cost comparison. If a certain product is considerably cheaper to make, then begin to look at the time involved in making the product and also look at the ways a recipe can be changed in order to make it as time-efficient as possible. Special diets can be a major factor in changing a health condition, losing weight, or just feeling better. Employing time- and money-saving efforts will help maintain a healthy lifestyle and less frustration while managing a special diet.

Glossary

allergy-free chocolate chips- chocolate chips containing no dairy, soy or gluten. Enjoy Life brand is an example of allergy-free chocolate chips.

allergy-free margarine- a high quality, organic margarine made without dariy, soy, nuts

amaranth flour- a flour made from the seed of the amaranth plant. Amaranth seeds are high in protein and are highly nutritious.

arrowroot powder-a natural thickener that can be used in place of cornstarch to thicken or in recipes

bean flour- a gluten-free flour made from grinding dry beans

chia seed flour- a gluten-free flour made from ground chia seeds. It is high in vitamins, minerals, fiber.

coconut flour- a flour made from finely ground coconut meat with most of the fat and moisture removed. This flour is low in carbohydrates, high in protein and fiber. May be used alone or in combination with other flours in baked goods.

coconut oil- an oil that is great substitute for butter or margarine. It stays solid at room temperature and has an extremely long shelf life. Use virgin organic coconut oil. This oil works well in breads and baked goods.

flaxseed- a seed with a nutty flavor. It can be used whole, toasted or sprouted; ground into meal; or pressed into oil. It is high in fiber and can be used as an egg replacer.

garbanzo bean flour- a gluten-free flour made from ground chick peas or garbanzo beans

ghee- butter clarified by cooking to evaporate out the water and to remove the milk solids

gluten-free flour mix- a mix of flours such as brown rice, bean, cornstarch, tapioca starch that do not include grains such as wheat, barley, rye or spelt. Gluten-free flour mixes usually contain a combination of a grain and starch and several different types of flours combined to equal the consistency of the flours containing gluten.

guar gum- a natural gum used as a thickener, emulsifier and stabilizer in food preparation. Commonly used in gluten free flour mixes.

milk alternative- a product such as almond, rice or coconut milk substituted for cow's milk to avoid allergies, lactose intolerance or to follow a vegan diet.

millet- a grain that is can be ground into flour and used in gluten-free flour recipes

nut butter- a nut ground to a creamy consistency, similar to peanut butter

potato flour- a flour made from potatoes but not to be confused with potato starch

potato starch- a fine white flour made from potatoes. It can be used in place of cornstarch.

quinoa- an ancient grain that has a high protein value and complete with all eight of the essential amino acids. It has a high source of vitamins and minerals, high in fiber and is gluten-free.

rice flour- a flour made from ground rice. Brown rice flour is more nutritious than white rice flour. It is gluten-free and commonly used in recipes.

sorghum flour- a flour ground from sorghum grain used in gluten-free flour mixes

tahini- nut butter made from sesame seeds

tapioca starch- a starch used as a thickener and stabilizer in food preparation. It is gluten-free and commonly used in gluten-free flour mixes. It can be used in place of cornstarch.

teff flour- a flour made from the tiny teff cereal grain. It is very nutritious and gluten-free

xanthan gum- a natural gum used as a thickener, emulsifier and stabilizer in food preparation. Commonly used in gluten free flour mixes.

Appendix A

FOOD SUBSTITUTIONS

BREAD ALTERNATIVES

Gluten-Free

Gluten-free bread

Gluten-free pancakes

Gluten-free crepes

Gluten-free waffles

Gluten-free crackers

Gluten-free pizza crust

Rice cakes

Tortillas (corn, spelt, rice, teff)

Gluten-Free Ready-Made Bread

English Muffins by Ener-G

Rice Bread by Cybros

Rice Bread by Ener-G

Tapioca Bread by Ener-G

Yeast Free Brown Rice Bread by Ener-G

Yeast Free White Rice Bread by Ener-G

Bagels by Enjoy Life

Bhutanese Red Rice Bread by Food For Life

Brown Rice Bread by Food For Life

Multi Seed Rice Bread by Food For Life

Raisin Pecan Bread by Food For Life

Rice Almond Bread by Food For Life

Rice Pecan Bread by Food For Life

White Rice Bread by Food For Life

Whole Grain Brown Rice Bread by Food For Life

Whole Grain Brown Rice Tortillas by Food For Life

Breads by Kinnikinnick's

Muffins by Kinnikinnick's

Bagels by Kinnikinnick's

Frozen Pizza Crust by Natures Hilights

Waffles by Van's

*Ready-Made Bread
(not gluten-free)*

Sprouted breads, bagels,

buns and tortillas by Alvarado St. Bakery

Sprouted breads, buns and tortillas Ezekiel Bread by Food For Life (regular or gluten-free varieties)

Sprouted breads, buns and tortillas Genesis Bread by Food For Life (regular or gluten-free varieties)

Whole grain breads, bagels, buns and tortillas by Rudi's

Bread Mixes

Gluten-Free Bread Mix by Bob's Red Mill

Gluten-Free Bread Mixes by Breads From Anna

Gluten-Free Bread Mixes by Gluten Free Pantry

Gluten-Free Pizza Mixes by Gluten Free Pantry

Favorite Sandwich Bread by Glutino (not dairy-free)

Gluten-Free Bread Mixes by Miss Roben's

Amazing Bread Mix by Pamela's Products

Think outside of the box. Eat meat without bread or bun. Serve sandwiches with a lettuce wrap. Peanut butter and jelly can be eaten on pancakes or waffles instead of bread.

CEREAL ALTERNATIVES
Gluten Free/ Dairy Free

Puffed Rice Cereal by Arrowhead Mills

Apple Raisin Walnut Granola by Bakery on Main

Extreme Fruit and Nut Granola by Bakery on Main

Nutty Cranberry Granola by Bakery on Main

Rainforest Granola by Bakery on Main

Brown Rice Crisps by Barbara's Bakery

Corn Flakes by Barbara's Bakery

Frosted Flakes by Barbara's Bakery

Rice Cereal (for babies) by Beechnut

Creamy Rice Hot Cereal by Bob's Red Mill

Cinnamon Crunch Granola Cereal by Enjoy Life

Cranapple Crunch Granola by Enjoy Life

Very Berry Granola Cereal by Enjoy Life

Amazon Frosted Flakes by Envirokids

Gorilla Munch by Envirokids

Koala Crisp by Envirokids

Peanut Butter Panda Puffs
by Envirokids

Corn Flakes Cereal by Erehwon

Crispy Brown Rice with Berries
Cereal by Erehwon

Rice Twice Cereal by Erehwon

Rice Cereal with Apples
by Gerber

Rice Cereal with Bananas
by Gerber

Single Grain Rice Cereal
by Gerber

Apple Cinnamon Cereal
by Glutino

Honey Nut Cereal by Glutino

Corn Crunch-Ems
by Health Valley

Rice Crunch-Ems
by Health Valley

Brown Rice Cereal
by Healthy Times

Belgian Chocolate Granola
Crunch by Lizi's

Lime and Ginger Granola
by Lizi's

Molasses and Pecan Granola
by Lizi's

Original Granola by Lizi's

Corn Bursts by Malt-O-Meal

Puffed Rice by Malt-O-Meal

Blue Corn Flakes by Nature's
Path

Honey'd Corn Flakes by
Nature's Path

Mesa Sunrise Flakes by Nature's
Path

Whole Grain Crispy Rice
by Nature's Path

Apple Cinnamon Perky O's
by Perky's

Frosted Perky O's by Perky's

Nutty Flax Cereal by Perky's

Original Perky O's by Perky's

Apple Almond Chia Goodness
by Ruth's Hemp Foods

Cranberry Ginger Chia
Goodness by Ruth's Hemp Foods

Original Chia Goodness
by Ruth's Hemp Foods

Pasta Alternatives (Gluten Free)

Elbows by Ancient Quinoa
Harvest (contains corn
and quinoa)

Spaghetti by Ancient
Quinoa Harvest (contains
corn and quinoa)

Rice Cheddar Pasta and Cheddar by Annie's (contains dairy)

Bean Threads (found in the ethnic section of the grocery store or specialty store)

Elbows by Bionaturae

Fusilli by Bionaturae

Penne by Bionaturae

Spaghetti by Bionaturae

Corn Elbows by DeBoles

Corn Spaghetti by DeBoles

Rice Angel Hair by DeBoles

Rice Fettuccine by DeBoles

Rice Lasagna by DeBoles

Rice Penne by DeBoles

Rice Spaghetti by DeBoles

Rice Spirals by DeBoles

Brown Rice Fusilli Pasta by Glutino

Brown Rice Macaroni by Glutino

Brown Rice Penne by Glutino

Brown Rice Spaghetti by Glutino

Penne Brown Rice Pasta by Lundburg

Rotini Brown Rice Pasta by Lundburg

Spaghetti Brown Rice Pasta by Lundburg

Miracle Noodle Shirataki Pasta*

Brown Rice Spaghetti by Mrs. Leeper's

Brown Rice Vegetable Twist by Mrs. Leeper's

Corn Elbows by Mrs. Leeper's

Corn Spaghetti by Mrs. Leeper's

Rice Alphabets by Mrs. Leeper's

Rice Shapes for Kids by Mrs. Leeper's

Rice Sticks (found in the ethnic section of the grocery store or specialty store)

Brown Rice Elbows by Tinkyada

Brown Rice Fettuccini by Tinkyada

Brown Rice Fusilli by Tinkyada

Brown Rice Grandshell by Tinkyada

Brown Rice Lasagna by Tinkyada

Brown Rice Littledreams by Tinkyada

Brown Rice Penne by Tinkyada

Brown Rice Shells by Tinkyada

Brown Rice Spaghetti
by Tinkyada

Brown Rice Spinach Spaghetti
by Tinkyada

Brown Rice Spiral by Tinkyada

Brown Rice Vegetable Spiral
by Tinkyada

*Miracle Noodle Shirataki Pasta
is from the root of a plant called
Konnyaku Imo. Order these noodles
atwww.miraclenoodle.com*

*Our favorite gluten-free pastas
are those made by Ancient Quinoa
Harvest (spaghetti), rice sticks,
Miracle Noodles and pastas by
Tinkyada.*

MILK ALTERNATIVES

*There are many alternatives to
milk depending on the use of the
milk. For drinking, there are
many rice, nut, and almond milks
that taste wonderful. Coconut
milk can be used for baking
or drinks, and powdered milk
alternative is great for travel and
long-term storage. The following
are a list of substitutions that can
be used for milk:*

Gluten- and Dairy-Free
Coconut milk, fresh

Edenblend Rice by Eden
Organic

Hemp Milk by Living Harvest

Almond Non-Dairy Beverage
(original and vanilla hazelnut)
by Pacific Foods

Pacific Rice (plain and vanilla)
by Pacific Foods

Pacific Ultra by Pacific Foods

Heartwise Rice Beverage
(original and vanilla) by Rice
Dream

Coconut Milk by So! Delicious
(good for drinking)

Rice Moo by Soy Good

Coconut Milk by Thai Kitchen
(good for evaporated milk or in
soups and casseroles)

Dairy-Free

Almond Breeze by Blue
Diamond

Ricemilk by Good Karma

Almond Dream
by Imagine Foods

Oat Beverage by Pacific Foods

Rice Beverage (carob, original
and vanilla) by Rice Dream

Rice drink (plain and vanilla)
by Westsoy

Rice Milk Powder by Better Than Milk

Soy Milk Powder (original and chocolate) by Better Than Milk

Dari-Free by Vance's Foods (potato based)

Coconut Milk Powder by Wilderness Family Naturals

Soy milk can also be used as a replacement for milk. Be aware that there is a controversy over the effects of soy on the thyroid and hormones in humans. Also be sure to check the soy milk to be sure it is dairy-free and also make sure it's gluten-free, if needed.

We use Dairi-Free powdered milk for many of our dairy needs. It does not always work well for cooking in casseroles or as a cream soup substitute. Almond Beverage by Pacific Foods and Coconut Milk by So! Delicious are other favorite milks that our family enjoys drinking. Coconut milk can also be substituted for many recipes calling for milk and it also has many beneficial health benefits.

BUTTER ALTERNATIVES

Applesauce —up to ¾ of the butter can be replaced with applesauce

Chia seeds — can replace some butter in recipes

Coconut Oil — virgin is less processed, but expeller pressed has less of a coconut flavor

Buttery Sticks by Earth Balance

Buttery Spread by Earth Balance

Ghee — also known as clarified butter and is 98% fat and the remaining is water

Safflower Oil Margarine by Hain's

Margarine — Be sure this contains non-hydrogenated oils! Smart Balance Light is a better choice; organic or all-natural margarines would be best choice

Non-dairy spread by Mother's Food Products, Inc.

Oil — non-hydrogenated is best, avoid low quality oils, 1/3 cup of oil will replace ½ cup of butter

Organic All Vegetable Shortening by Spectrum

½ cup of pitted prunes pureed with ¼ cup water can replace up to ¾ of the butter in a recipe

If you need to be gluten, soy and dairy free the best choices are non-hydrogenated oil such as olive, grapeseed, sunflower, canola, sesame, macadamia, hazelnut or coconut oils or Shortening by Spectrum.

Cheese Alternatives

Pimento Cheese (see recipe instructions in recipe section)

Cheese Sauce
by Road's End Organics

Vegan Soymage (mozzarella, yellow American, Parmesan, low -fat Parmesan, soy cream cheese) by Soyco, Galaxy Foods

Vegan Chunk Line (mozzarella, cheddar, jalapeño, Italian herb) by Soyco, Galaxy Foods

ICE CREAM ALTERNATIVES

Homemade ice cream or sorbet

Luna & Larry's Coconut Bliss (8 flavors)

Purely Decadent coconut ice-creams by Turtle Mountain (5 flavors)

Rice Dream, vanilla
(Rice Dream)

Sharon's Sorbet (2 flavors)

Sorbet (dairy-free)

Coldstone Creamery
(dairy –free sorbets)

PEANUT BUTTER ALTERNATIVES

Almond butter

Cashew butter

Hazelnut butter

Macadamia nut butter

Soy butter

Sunflower butter

Many different types of nuts can be ground to make nut butters. Sunflower butter can be used if there is a tree nut or peanut allergy. See the recipe section to make your own nut butter.

SUGAR ALTERNATIVES

Agave nectar

Blackstrap molasses

Honey

Maple syrup

Molasses

Stevia

Xylitol

CHIPS, PRETZELS, AND SNACKS

Tortilla Chips by Bearitos

Brown Rice Snaps
by Edward & Sons

Saltines by Ener-G

Wylde Pretzels by Ener-G

Frito's by Frito Lay

Lay's Original by Frito Lay

Ruffles Original by Frito Lay

Tostitos Unflavored Tortilla
Chips by Frito Lay

Tortilla Chips
by Garden of Eatin'

Pretzels (all varieties) by Glutino

Crackers (all varieties)
by Mary's Gone Crackers

Sticks and Twigs (pretzels)
by Mary's Gone Crackers

Original Cracklebread
by Natural Nectar

Rice Thins by Sesmark

Terra Chips by Terra

This is a small list and does not include most varieties of chips or crackers. Check the labels of chips to be sure they are labeled gluten-free and/or dairy free. Most potato chips and tortilla chips without flavorings may be gluten-free and dairy-free. Many varieties of cheese flavored chips found in a health food store or health food section of a store are gluten-free but not dairy-free. Be sure to avoid all products containing partially hydrogenated or hydrogenated oils and artificial colors and flavorings. Eat a limited amount of processed snack foods.

COOKIES

The following brands manufacture many types of gluten-free and/or dairy-free cookies:

Andean

Arico

Cherry

Enjoy Life

Envirokids

Glutino

Jennie

Jo-sef

Kinnikinnick

Mary's Gone Crackers

Midel

Nana

There are many other companies that produce gluten-free or dairy-free cookies. Check the labels of each product to be sure they do not contain gluten or dairy. Envirokids Vanilla Animal Cookies and cookies from Glutino are our favorites.

SNACK IDEAS

Prepared foods

applesauce

banana chips

dried fruit

fruit leather

guacamole

juice popsicles

popcorn

pretzels

rice crackers

salsa

smoothies

trail mix

Fresh fruit

apples

bananas

blueberries

cantaloupe

cherries

fruit bits

grapes

honeydew

kiwis

mandarin oranges

mangos

oranges

peaches

pears

pineapple

plums

prunes

raisins   strawberries

watermelon slices

Fresh vegetables

broccoli pieces

carrot sticks

cauliflower pieces

celery sticks

cucumber slices

fresh green beans

fresh peas

frozen peas

green peppers

kohlrabi

radishes

Protein-rich snacks

nuts

seeds

hard boiled egg

"ants on a log" (spread peanut butter on pieces of celery; add raisins)

Appendix B

WHAT'S IN THE PANTRY

Looking at all the steps and procedures in this book may seem overwhelming to start at first. Start slow and don't try to change everything at once. I do use most of the money and time saving methods at some point during the year. Which methods I use vary greatly by the time of year, my work schedule, my children's activities and travel plans. I tend to make more mixes in the winter and home grown foods in the summer. Sometimes I make a mix. Sometimes I use fresh or home grown fruits and vegetables. Sometimes I purchase items on sale, if it is cheaper than making it from scratch. So what's in my pantry? Let's take a look:

Pantry:

Pasta, gluten-free (purchased on sale half price)

Cocoa

Chia seeds

Sunflower seeds

Pumpkin seeds

Dried fruit

Peanuts

Ghee

Coconut oil

Spices

Dried beans and lentils

Quinoa

Brown rice (not instant)

Muffin mix, gluten-free

Wheat flour (King Arthur brand)

Oatmeal

Cream soup substitute mix, dairy-free (homemade, make several times a year)

Pancake mix, gluten-free (homemade, make several times a year)

In-a-jar cookie mix, gluten-free

In-a-jar cake mix, gluten-free

Vinegar (balsamic and white distilled)

Oil (olive, grapeseed, sunflower... non-hydrogenated brands)

Popcorn

Cornstarch

Powdered sugar (C & H brand)

Brown sugar (C & H brand)

Organic sugar

Salt (sea salt and Celtic sea salt)

Baking powder (aluminum free)

Baking soda

Xanthan gum

Brown rice flour

Corn meal

Millet flour

Coconut flour

Quinoa flour

Chia flour

Sorghum flour

Garbanzo bean flour

Tapioca starch

Cornstarch

All purpose gluten-free flour

Kombucha

Bulk Items Homemade or Purchased on Sale:

Pizza crust mix (cheaper than homemade)

Gluten-free bread mix (cheaper than homemade)

Pasta sauce

Sunflower butter

Rice cakes

Cold cereal

Miracle noodles

Salsa (home grown tomatoes made into salsa to can)

Relish (home grown zucchini to make into relish to can)

Refrigerator:

Italian dressing mix (make once a year or less)

Ranch dressing mix (make once a year or less)

Pizza seasoning mix (make once a year or less)

Flax seed

Flax meal (for making egg alternative)

Bread, gluten-free

Fresh fruit, seasonal

Fresh vegetables, seasonal

Deli lunchmeat

Deli cheese

Coconut milk (purchased on sale at half price)

Cow's milk, organic (purchased on sale)

Butter

Mayonnaise, gluten-free (purchased on sale)

Ketchup, gluten-free, organic (purchased on sale)

Chocolate chips, gluten-free and dairy-free (purchased on sale)

Ah!Laska chocolate sauce, gluten-free and dairy-free (purchased on sale)

Jam (homemade)

Sunflower butter (purchased on sale in bulk)

Leftovers and food to be used in Method 6 -"Piggy-Back Cooking"

Freezer:

Bacon, cooked (purchased on sale then oven baked)

Corndogs (homemade)

Chicken, cooked and shredded

Turkey, cooked and diced

Hamburger patty, cooked

Lunchmeat (purchased on sale)

Sausages, cooked (homemade)

Pancakes (homemade)

Waffles (purchased for a trip, we don't purchase these often)

Deep Freezer:

Gluten-free cookies (homemade)

Gluten-free cake (homemade)

Chicken broth (homemade)

Dairy-free ice cream (purchased with a coupon)

Syrup (homemade, tapped from our birch tree)

Coconut water (extracted from a young coconut)

Deer meat, (from a deer we received for free from a friend)

Hamburger (packaged in pound packages, purchased from ¼ of a grass fed cow)

Cheese (purchased on sale $1 for 8 oz.)

Frozen fruit (purchased on sale)

Frozen vegetables (purchased on sale)

Tomatoes (home grown, sliced in half, then frozen)

Frozen pizza and fish sticks (purchased on sale...for emergencies only as we don't eat these often)

The Recipes

A pinch..................................1/8 tablespoon or less

3 teaspoons............................1 tablespoon

4 tablespoons.........................¼ cup

5 ⅓ tablespoons.....................⅓ cup

8 tablespoons.........................½ cup

10 ⅔ tablespoons...................⅔ cup

12 tablespoons.......................¾ cup

16 tablespoons.......................1 cup

2 cups....................................1 pint

4 cups....................................1 quart

4 quarts.................................1 gallon

8 quarts.................................1 peck

4 pecks..................................1 bushel

16 ounces..............................1 pound

32 ounces..............................1 quart

1 ounce liquid.......................2 tablespoons

8 ounces liquid......................1 cup

ABBREVIATIONS

1 tablespoon = 1 Tbsp. = 1 T.

1 teaspoon = 1 tsp. = 1 t.

1 cup = 1 c.

1 quart = 1 qt.

1 ounce = 1 oz.

Alternatives

GLUTEN-FREE FLOUR ALTERNATIVES

When using gluten-free flour as an alternative to wheat flour, a mix of several ingredients must be made in order to create a similar consistency to wheat flour. The recipes in this section can be mixed ahead of time and stored in a container with a tight-fitting lid or a large sealed bag. Use Method 5—Bulk Prepared Mixes in Chapter 4, "Planning How to Cook" to save time in preparation of the gluten-free flour mixes. You can also save money by preparing your own gluten-free flour mixes (see Chapter 6, "Store Bought vs. Homemade").

When cooking with gluten-free flours, add 1 teaspoon of xanthan gum or guar gum to each cup of mix used in breads and baked goods. Less can be used if you're making cakes or cookies. I have found that xanthan gum is much more expensive than guar gum but has a better quality when cooking. Sometimes xanthan gum is not needed for a particular recipe. All of the ingredients for the flour mixes and the xanthan gum can be purchased at a health food store, on the internet, or in a health food section of a local grocery store.

Arrowroot starch or potato starch can be substituted for cornstarch in these mixes if you have a corn sensitivity; however, it may make the product crumbly, and arrowroot starch is more expensive than cornstarch.

The following three recipes were taken from *The Gluten-Free Gourmet Makes Dessert* by Bette Hagman. I feel that they are the best quality and least expensive of all flour mixes.

Bette Hagman's Light Bean Flour Mix

Garfava flour	1 part	or 1 cup
Tapioca starch	1 part	or 1 cup
Cornstarch	1 part	or 1 cup

I use this mix primarily for bread making, but it also works well in other baked goods. I feel that it gives sweet baked goods too bitter a flavor.

Bette Hagman's Dark Bean Flour Mix

Garfava flour	2 parts	or	⅔ cup
Sorghum flour	1 part	or	⅓ cup
Tapioca starch	3 parts	or	1 cup
Cornstarch	3 parts	or	1 cup

I use this mix primarily for bread making, but it also works well in other baked goods. I often substitute garbanzo bean flour for garfava flour, depending on the availability in our local grocery stores. The garbanzo bean flour is usually less expensive than garfava flour.

Bette Hagman's Featherlight Flour Mix

Rice flour	3 parts	or	1 cup
Tapioca flour	3 parts	or	1 cup
Cornstarch	3 parts	or	1 cup
Potato flour	1 teaspoon per cup		

I use this mix for cakes, cookies, brownies, muffins, and breads. It tastes best in sweet-tasting baked goods. I do not use the potato flour in this mix because it is not readily available in our area grocery stores; in my experience, the mix works fine without it.

The following is a general all-purpose mix that I developed that can be used with bread or other baked goods. I developed this flour when I accidentally ran out of rice flour and substituted part of the rice flour with bean flour. This mix is our favorite for breads.

Beans and Rice Mix

Rice flour	½ part	or	½ cup
Garbanzo bean flour	½ part	or	½ cup
Tapioca flour	1 part	or	1 cup
Cornstarch	1 part	or	1 cup

The following four recipes were taken from the Living Without web site at www.livingwithout.com. Living Without is a magazine for people who have allergies and food sensitivities. It is an excellent resource. I highly recommend subscribing to the magazine and using its web site as a reference.

All-Purpose Flour Blend

Rice flour	½ part	or	½ cup
Tapioca flour	¼ part	or	¼ cup
Cornstarch	¼ part	or	¼ cup

High-Fiber Flour Blend

1 cup brown rice flour or sorghum flour
1/2 cup teff flour (preferably light)
1/2 cup millet flour or Montina® flour
2/3 cup tapioca starch/flour
1/3 cup cornstarch or potato starch

This high-fiber blend works for breads, pancakes, snack bars, and cookies that contain chocolate, warm spices, raisins, or fruits. It is not suited to delicately flavored recipes such as sugar cookies, crepes, cream puffs, birthday cakes, or cupcakes.

High-Protein Flour Blend

1 1/4 cups bean flour (your choice), chickpea flour, or soy flour
1 cup arrowroot starch, cornstarch, or potato starch
1 cup tapioca starch/flour
1 cup white rice flour or brown rice flour

This nutritious blend works best in baked goods that require elasticity, such as wraps and pie crusts.

Self-Rising Flour Blend

1 1/4 cups white sorghum flour

1 1/4 cups white rice flour

1/2 cup tapioca starch/flour

2 teaspoons xanthan gum or guar gum

4 teaspoons baking powder

1/2 teaspoon salt

Use this blend for muffins, scones, cakes, cupcakes, or any recipe that uses baking powder for leavening.

MILK ALTERNATIVES

Milk alternatives are typically used in place of cow's milk for a dairy allergy or intolerance. There are many alternatives to milk, depending on the use. For drinking, many rice, nut, and almond milks taste wonderful. Coconut milk can be used for baking (beverage or canned) or for drinking (beverage), and powdered milk alternative is great for travel and long-term storage.

Many milk alternatives can be purchased at the grocery store, but they can be quite costly. For example, almond milk currently runs about $3.50 per quart, or $14.00 per gallon, and beverage coconut milk is about $4.20 per half gallon, or $8.40 per gallon. The following are recipes that can be used in lieu of milk alternatives from the store.

Nut Milks

    1 c. raw nuts of choice (see below)

    2–4 c. water

    1–2 T. agave nectar, maple syrup, or honey

    pinch of salt

Combine nuts, water, agave nectar, and salt in a blender. Blend on high until the nuts are completely broken down. Pour milk through strainer, nut bag, or coffee filter and squeeze as much of the liquid out as possible. Reserve the liquid and use the nut milk to drink or for any recipe calling for milk or milk alternative.

Nut milks can also be used to make yogurt. They also can be frozen. Use the leftover pulp in smoothies, hummus, or breads, or tossed on cereal, vegetables, or rice. The pulp can also be frozen. Making your own nut milk will save about $1.00 per quart ($4.00 per gallon), takes only a few minutes to make, and tastes great!

Almond Milk

Soak almonds in filtered water for at least 12 hours in the refrigerator. Drain the water. Add one cup of pre-soaked almonds to the recipe above.

Brazil Nut Milk

One cup raw Brazil nuts added to the nut milk recipe above. Brazil nuts are high in selenium. Selenium is a powerful antioxidant that helps protect against disease and that slows the aging process and boosts the immune system.

Hazelnut, Pecan, Walnut, Cashew, or Macadamia Nut Milk

Use one cup of raw nuts added to the recipe above.

Hemp Seed Milk

Use 3/4 cup of raw hemp seeds in lieu of raw nuts to the recipe above.

Quick Nut Milk

    2 c. purified water
    2 T. nut butter (almond, cashew, macadamia, etc.)
    1 T. agave nectar, maple syrup, or honey
    pinch of salt

Combine water, nut butter, and sweetener in a blender. Blend on high until smooth.

Rice Milk

    1 c. rice, cooked
    4 c. water, filtered
    2 T. agave nectar, maple syrup, or honey

Combine rice, water, and sweetener in a blender. Blend on high until the rice is completely broken down. Pour milk through strainer, nut bag, or coffee filter and squeeze as much of the liquid out as possible. Reserve the liquid and use the rice milk to drink or for any recipe calling for milk or milk alternative.

Coconut Milk Drink

    1 can coconut milk
    2 c. water
    1 T. vanilla

Combine canned coconut milk, water, and vanilla in a blender. Blend on high until well mixed. If the mixture is too thick, add more water. Add a small amount of agave nectar or honey to sweeten if needed. Drink or use immediately, or refrigerate.

Fresh Coconut Milk Drink

    1 c. shredded coconut meat
    2 c. water
    1 T. agave nectar, maple syrup, or honey

Use an ice pick and hammer to tap a hole in a coconut.* Remove the liquid from the inside of the coconut.** Next, crack open the coconut and remove the coconut meat (the inside flesh) from the coconut or use unsweetened shredded coconut from a package. Combine coconut, water, and sweetener in a blender. Blend on high until well mixed. Strain the liquid from the mixture if the shredded coconut is still present. Drink or use immediately, or refrigerate.

*A mature or young coconut can be used. A mature coconut is brown on the outside, whereas a young coconut is white on the outside. I use young coconuts because they are easier to tap into and to crack open.

**The liquid from the inside of the coconut can be reserved and used for recipes such as coconut kefir or even electrolyte drinks.

Note: This recipe is not cheaper or easier than buying coconut milk. The benefits of this recipe is that the milk can be made fresh and that there are no added ingredients.

EGG ALTERNATIVES

Egg alternatives are used for those having an allergy or intolerance to eggs. Some individuals are intolerant to sulfur, a component of eggs. Some individuals who cannot tolerate chicken eggs may be able to tolerate quail or duck eggs. Be sure to check your state laws to see if either quail or duck eggs are legal to sell or purchase. Some of the egg alternatives listed below work better than others. I have found that the egg-free egg alternatives do not work as well in baking as the alternatives containing eggs. In our household, we use the flaxseed meal or ground chia seeds (1 T.) plus water (3 T.) combination for egg-free cooking. That combination works well for breads and cakes. Cooking times may vary if using an egg alternative, and the baked product may not have the same texture or height of the original recipe.

Use any of the following combinations to replace 1 egg:

Egg-Free:

Egg substitute (Ener-G Foods; contains potato)

Egg substitute (Bob's Red Mill)

1 tablespoon flaxseed meal + 3 tablespoons water blended smooth; let sit 5 min.

1 tablespoon ground chia seeds + 3 tablespoons water blended smooth; let sit 5 min.

1 tablespoon tahini + 3 tablespoons liquid

1 tablespoon garbanzo flour + 1 tablespoon oil

1 tablespoon arrowroot powder + 3 tablespoons liquid

1 teaspoon yeast dissolved in 1/4 cup warm water

1 1/2 tablespoons water + 1 1/2 tablespoons oil + 1 teaspoon baking powder

1 packet gelatin + 2 tablespoons warm water (don't mix until ready to use)

1 packet gelatin + 1 cup boiling water (Use 3 tablespoons for every egg needed.)

1 tablespoon soy lecithin granules + 3 tablespoons liquid

1 tablespoon arrowroot powder + 3 tablespoons liquid

1 teaspoon baking powder + 1 tablespoon water + 1 tablespoon vinegar

1 tablespoon apricot puree

1/3 cup applesauce (for muffins, brownies, and cakes)

1/3 cup pumpkin puree (for pies and baking)

½ mashed banana (for quick breads, muffins, breads, and pancakes)

Not Egg-Free:

2 egg yolks + 1 tablespoon cold water

3 ½ tablespoons thawed frozen egg

2 ½ tablespoons powdered whole egg + 2 1/2 tablespoons water

2 large egg whites + 1 tablespoon nonfat milk powder + 1 teaspoon canola oil

quail egg

duck egg

Peanut Butter Alternatives

Many types of nuts and seeds can be ground to make nut butters, including almonds, cashews, hazelnuts, macadamia nuts, sunflower or sesame seeds. Try the recipe below to make your own nut butter.

Nut Butter

  1 ½ c. nuts or seeds (almond, macadamia, cashew, etc.)

    2 T. oil

Dash of salt (optional)

Place nuts in a blender or food processor. Blend or process for one minute, turning the machine off every ten seconds, until the nuts have turned into a thick paste. Add oil slowly, starting with one tablespoon, to get clumping action started. Turn the machine off every 30 seconds during this final stage, which may take about three minutes.

Use roasted or unroasted nuts and seeds. If you leave the skins on, you'll have a butter richer in fiber and nutrition. This is much cheaper than purchasing nut butters from the store, but sometimes the texture is not as smooth.

Appetizers and Snacks

Easy Salsa

12 medium tomatoes
1 large white onion
1 bunch cilantro (1–1 ½ cups)
3–6 large jalapeno peppers
1 bunch green onions

Chop vegetables; mix and refrigerate. This salsa is best fresh. It can be frozen but will be very runny when thawed.

Bean and Salsa Dip

1 c. salsa, or more
15 oz. refried beans

Heat beans on low on stovetop until soft, about 5 minutes. Add salsa. Serve with tortilla chips.

Guacamole

2–3 large tomatoes (1 ½ cups)
¼ c. finely chopped onion
¼ c. chopped fresh cilantro
1 ½ T. fresh lime juice
½ t. salt
2 ripe avocados, peeled and mashed

Combine all ingredients. Mix gently. Let stand 10 minutes to allow flavors to blend. Serve with tortilla chips or over tacos, or top your favorite Mexican dish.

Hummus

   2 c. chickpeas (garbanzo beans), cooked
   4 T. tahini*
   2 T. lemon juice
   1 T. olive oil
   2 t. fresh parsley
   2 cloves pressed garlic
   1 t. ground cumin
   4 oz. roasted red peppers (optional)

Drain chickpeas if using canned. Blend in the blender or food processor. Mix the garlic, lemon juice, and tahini together and add to blender or food processor. Add remaining ingredients and puree; chill and serve. Serve with raw veggies or corn chips or use as a spread on a sandwich.

If you do not have tahini on hand, use cashew butter or sunflower butter instead or puree sesame seeds in a food processor with a little water to make a paste.

Puppy Chow

   7 ½ c. gluten-free cereal *(Rice or Corn Crunch Ems, Gorilla Munch, any bland-flavored gluten-free cereal)*
   1 c. allergy-free chocolate chips
   ¼ c. peanut butter or favorite nut butter
   1 c. powdered sugar

In a heavy 3-quart saucepan, melt chocolate over low heat until completely melted. Remove from heat. Stir in peanut butter. Add cereal. Place powdered sugar in 2-gallon zipper plastic bag. Add cereal mixture to sugar and close bag. Gently toss until evenly coated. Store in airtight container in refrigerator.

I adapted this recipe from a Crispix cereal box recipe. This recipe does contain sugar, so have this only occasionally. Quick and easy!

Honey Popcorn Crunch

    1/3 c. melted butter, ghee, or allergy-free margarine

    ½ c. honey

    6 quarts popcorn, popped

    1 c. nuts (optional)

Blend honey and butter; heat until well blended. In a separate container, combine the popcorn and nuts. Pour honey-butter blend over popcorn-nut mixture and mix well. Spread over greased cookie sheet in a thin layer. Bake at 350 degrees for 2–5 minutes or until crisp.

Gluten-Free Snack Mix

    6 T. butter, ghee, or allergy-free margarine

    2 T. allergy-free Worcestershire sauce

    3 c. Rice Crunch Ems

    3 c. puffed corn

    3 c. Corn Crunch Ems

    3 c. puffed rice

  1 ½ t. garlic powder

    ⅛ t. cayenne pepper

Melt butter; add seasonings. Toss mixture with cereals. Bake at 250 degrees for 1 hour, stirring every 15 minutes.

Gluten-free pretzels, nuts, popcorn, other cereals, or whatever you want can be substituted for the puffed corn, puffed rice, Corn Crunch Ems, and Rice Crunch Ems; total should be 12 cups.

Trail Mix

raisins	nuts	allergy-free chocolate chips
dried fruit	coconut	gluten-free pretzels
popcorn	seeds	allergy-free cold cereal

Mix equal amounts of any of the above ingredients in an airtight container or bag.

You can use any combination of foods. I just use whatever is in my pantry. Sometimes it is as simple as dried fruit and nuts.

Flavored Popcorn

popcorn, air popped or pan popped
Olive oil spray (for air-popped corn)

Toppings, choose one of the following:

chili powder	onion powder
garlic powder	cinnamon
taco seasoning	Italian seasoning

Place warm popcorn in an airtight container. Spray lightly with oil spray if the popcorn is air popped. Sprinkle 2 t. of topping for every 1/2 cup *un*popped popcorn over cooked popcorn. Seal container and shake well. Serve warm.

Popcorn can be difficult to digest or may aggravate the intestines, so limit popcorn consumption in people with digestive problems.

Ranch Popcorn

2 t. ranch dressing mix (see p. 98) or ranch seasoning
1 T. oil (may use less)
2–3 quarts popped popcorn

Combine ranch dressing mix or ranch seasoning with the oil. Place popcorn in airtight container with a lid. Add oil mixture and shake well. Serve immediately.

Italian Popcorn

　2　t. Italian dressing mix (see p. 101) or Italian seasoning

　1　T. oil, may use less oil

2-3　quarts of popped popcorn

Combine Italian dressing mix or Italian seasoning with the oil. Place popcorn in airtight container with a lid. Add oil mixture and shake well. Serve immediately.

Carmel Corn

2–3　quarts popped popcorn

　½　c. water

　½　c. molasses

　1　c. sugar

　½　t. vinegar (gluten-free)

　½　t. soda

　1　T. butter, ghee, or allergy-free margarine

Combine water, molasses, sugar, vinegar, and butter and boil to 270 degrees or until the mixture cracks in cold water. Remove from heat and add soda. Stir well and pour over popcorn; mix.

This recipe is high in sugar, so do not eat this often.

Fruit Salsa

　3　apples, coarsely chopped

　2　c. strawberries, diced, or raspberries or a mix of the two

　3　kiwi, peeled and diced

　2　T. orange juice

　2　T. apricot jam

Combine fruit in a bowl. Combine juice and jam. Stir juice and jam mixture gently into fruit mixture. Serve with tortilla chips.

Gluten-Free Beef Jerky

   3 T. garlic powder
2 ½ T. black pepper
   ½ c. brown sugar
   1 t. garlic salt
   7 cloves garlic
     red pepper to taste
   1 t. onion powder
   2 T. gluten-free Worcestershire sauce
  12 oz. Bragg's Liquid Aminos or gluten-free soy sauce
   3 pounds rump roast, cut with grain and trimmed of fat

Combine all ingredients except meat. Slice the meat thinly (the meat can partially be frozen first). Place the meat in a large pan; pour the marinade over the top and soak for at least 15 minutes. Turn over meat slices after 8 minutes. Place the meat on the racks of a dehydrator. Do not overlap meat. Dry until jerky rips when bent. Slices should be turned over halfway through dehydrating to ensure even drying.

Ants on a Log

   5 celery stalks
   ½ c. peanut butter or other nut butter
     raisins

Cut celery stalks into thirds. Spread centers of celery with peanut butter. Sprinkle with raisins.

Baked Pumpkin Seeds

Remove contents from a pumpkin. Separate seeds from pulp and string, and rinse seeds. Place seeds in a single layer on ungreased baking sheet. Bake in preheated 325 degree oven for 15–20 minutes until dry and lightly brown, or for 30–40 minutes if you like them crispy. Season with sea salt if desired.

Beverages

Fruit Spritzer

  12 oz. unsweetened frozen juice concentrate

  36 oz. club soda

Mix frozen juice concentrate according to directions on the can, substituting club soda for water. Serve immediately.

Use this in place of soda. For a single serving, use 2 oz. juice concentrate combined with 6 oz. club soda.

Watermelon Slushes

  4 c. watermelon (about 1/4 medium), seeds removed

  3 T. fresh lime juice

  ⅔ c. orange juice

  2 quarts sparkling water

Combine watermelon, lime juice, and orange juice in blender until smooth. Combine mixture with sparkling water. Serves 3–4.

Fruit Cooler

  3 c. lemonade
  3 c. limeade
  3 c. fruit juice
  2 quarts sparkling water

Freeze the lemonade, limeade, and juice separately into ice cube trays. Place a mix of ice cubes in a cup and top with sparkling water when ready to serve. Garnish with lemon or lime slices.

Iced Tea

  6 t. tea leaves or tea and herbs and spices
  1 quart cold water

Combine tea and water in a quart jar. Cap the jar and shake it or stir leaves with a spoon for a moment. Leave the jar in the refrigerator for at least 12 hours. Strain tea and sweeten to taste with sugar, agave nectar, honey, or other sweetener. Add lemon, lime, or orange slices as the tea flavor dictates.

Basic Smoothie

  1 c. milk or milk alternative
  1 c. fruit juice
  1 c. fruit

Combine all ingredients in a blender. Puree until well mixed. Serve immediately.

Ideas for smoothies (choose one from each column):

almond milk	apple-raspberry juice	raspberries
coconut milk*	apple-cherry juice	strawberries
DariFree milk	orange juice	mango
rice milk	grape juice	blueberries
		pineapple
		peaches

*Use ¼ c. canned coconut milk or 1 c. So Delicious brand coconut milk.

Blueberry Smoothie

2 c. almond milk or milk alternative

1   banana

1/2 c. blueberries

Combine all ingredients in a blender. Puree until well mixed. Serve immediately.

Raspberry Smoothie

1 c. milk alternative

1 c. orange juice

1 c. raspberries

Combine all ingredients in a blender. Puree until well mixed. Serve immediately.

Dairy-Free Eggnog

3/4 canned coconut milk*

3 eggs, slightly beaten

1/2 c. granulated sugar

1/2 T. salt

3 c. milk alternative, liquid

1/2 t. vanilla

In a medium saucepan, combine eggs, sugar, and salt. Stir in coconut milk and milk alternative and cook on low to medium heat until the mixture coats a spoon (about 10 minutes). Stir constantly to prevent scorching. Remove from heat and add vanlla. Serve immediately or refrigerate. This recipe can be frozen.

* For a substitute, combine 1 cup of milk alternative powder (such as DariFree) and 3/4 cup hot water in a blender or mix 1 cup powdered milk and 1/2 cup water.

This recipe is high in sugar but is dairy free and lacks the corn syrup, additives, and preservatives of commercial eggnog.

Condiments

Ranch Dressing Mix

Small Batch		Large Batch
5	gluten-free rice crackers	15
½ c.	dry minced parsley flakes	1½ c.
2 T.	dry minced onions	½ c.
½ T.	dill weed	2 T.
1 T.	onion salt	¼ c.
1 T.	garlic salt	¼ c.
1 T.	onion powder	¼ c.
1 T.	garlic powder	¼ c.

Put crackers through blender on high speed until powdered. Add parsley, minced onions, and dill weed. Blend again until powdered. Dump into bowl. Stir in onion salt, garlic salt, onion powder, and garlic powder. Put into container with tight-fitting lid. Store at room temperature or in refrigerator for up to one year. Serving size is 1 T. Large batch makes 42 servings.

Make the large batch of this recipe and it will last up to one year. Less time is spent shopping in the store, and you always have ingredients for ranch dressing and ranch dip on hand at all times. This recipe will cost less than buying packets at the store. In addition, the ingredients that are in the mix can be regulated.

This recipe is the closest I could find to Hidden Valley Ranch dressing mix. It is very convenient, and I used it many years before our allergy-free days.

Dairy-Free Ranch Dressing

    1 T. ranch dressing mix
    ½ c. allergy-free mayonnaise
    ½ c. milk alternative

Combine all ingredients in a bowl and whisk together. Serve immediately or store in refrigerator up to 1 week.

Dairy-Free Ranch Dip

    1 T. ranch dressing mix
    1 c. allergy-free mayonnaise
    1 T. DariFree milk

Combine all ingredients in a bowl and whisk together. Serve
immediately or store in refrigerator up to one week.

Cherry Vinaigrette

    ½ c. frozen cherry juice concentrate
    ½ c. oil
    3 T. apple cider vinegar (Bragg's brand is best)
       pepper to taste

Blend ingredients in a blender or shake in a jar with a tight lid to
combine. Serve over a bed of lettuce. Can top with pine nuts, oranges,
red grapes, marinated onions, or blue cheese (if allowed in the diet), or
any combination.

Creamy Honey Mustard Vinaigrette

    ¼ c. allergy-free mayonnaise
    2 T. honey
    2 T. dry mustard
    ¼ t. salt
    2 t. apple cider vinegar (Bragg's is best)

Combine mayonnaise, honey, mustard, and salt and whisk until
well blended. Add vinegar and whisk until well blended. Cover and
refrigerate until ready to use. Can store covered up to 2 weeks.

Strawberry Vinaigrette

1 pint strawberries
½ c. rice wine vinegar
2 T. lemon juice
1 ½ t. canola oil
2 T. honey
¼ t. pepper
¼ t. salt

In a blender, combine strawberries, vinegar, lemon juice, oil, and honey until well blended. Season with salt and pepper to taste.

Grenadine

2 c. pomegranate juice
2 c. granulated sugar

Bring pomegranate juice to a boil; reduce heat to simmer. Add sugar. Stir continuously until all the sugar is dissolved. Store up to 2 weeks in the refrigerator. This can be frozen.

Grenadine is a cherry-type syrup often used in beverages such as grenadine and Coke (Roy Rogers cocktails) and nonalcoholic Shirley Temples. Cherries can also be soaked in grenadine to give them a bright red color to be used in cakes and cooking.

Italian Dressing Mix

Small Batch	Large Batch
¼ c. garlic salt	1 c.
2 ½ T. dried parsley flakes	¾ c.
1 t. garlic powder	4 t.
½ t. onion powder	2 t.
2 T. oregano	½ c.
1 t. basil	4 t.
1 t. paprika	4 t.
1 t. celery seeds	4 t.
2 T. sugar	½ c.
½ t. pepper	2 t.

Combine all ingredients. Put into container with tight-fitting lid. Store at room temperature or in refrigerator for up to one year. Use 1 1/2 tablespoons to replace a .6 oz. Italian dressing packet mix.

Make the large batch of this recipe and it will last up to one year. Less time is spent shopping in the store, and you always have ingredients for ranch dressing on hand at all times. This recipe will cost less than buying packets at the store. In addition, the ingredients that are in the mix can be regulated.

Italian Dressing

1–1½ T. Italian dressing mix
   ¼ c. vinegar
   3 T. water
   3/4 c. oil

Mix vinegar and water in a cruet, blender, or container with a lid. Add seasoning mix. Shake vigorously or blend well. Add oil and shake or blend again. Serve. This will store at room temperature for several weeks.

I use apple cider vinegar or balsamic vinegar for the vinegar, but any vinegar will work. I also use olive oil or grapeseed oil for the oil, but any oil will work.

Freezer Spaghetti Sauce

  3 c. onions
  ¾ c. oil
  4 cloves garlic
  5 quarts tomato juice, freshly juiced or canned
 12 oz. tomato paste
  ¼ c. sugar
  2 T. salt
  2 t. pepper
  2 T. oregano leaves
  2 t. basil leaves
  4 bay leaves

Combine all ingredients and cook slowly while stirring for 45 minutes to 1 hour or longer. Let sauce cool, remove bay leaves, and freeze.

To use: Thaw sauce overnight in the refrigerator or in a container with warm water. Warm the sauce on the stove and add 1–2 T. of cornstarch, tapioca starch, arrowroot powder, or other thickener.

This recipe is from my friend Laura Kuntz.

Taco Sauce

Small Batch		Large Batch
½ c.	tomato paste	3 c.
1 t.	chili powder	2 T.
½ t.	salt	1 T.
⅛ t.	cayenne pepper	1 T.
1	dash hot pepper sauce	½ t.
¾ c.	water	5 c.
3 T.	apple cider vinegar	1 c.
1 ½ T.	agave nectar or honey	½ c.

Combine all ingredients in a saucepot and bring to a boil. Reduce heat and simmer until thick, stirring frequently. Serve immediately or freeze.

Taco Seasoning Mix

Small Batch		Large batch
1 T.	chili powder	¾ c.
¼ t.	garlic powder	1 T.
¼ t.	onion powder	1 T.
¼ t.	crushed red pepper flakes	1 T.
¼ t.	dried oregano	1 T
½ t.	paprika	2 T.
½ t.	ground cumin	2 T.
1 t.	salt	¼ c.
1 t.	black pepper	¼ c.

Combine all ingredients and put into container with tight-fitting lid. Store at room temperature or in refrigerator for up to one year. One 1.25 oz. store-bought packet equals 2 1/2 tablespoons of this mix.

Enchilada Sauce

Small Batch		Large Batch
2 T.	chili powder	½ c.
1 ½ t.	olive oil	2 T.
1 c.	chicken broth	4 c.
1 t.	garlic salt	4 t.
½ T.	cornstarch	2 T.
1 c.	water	4 c.
1 c.	tomato sauce	4 c.

In a medium heated saucepot, brown chili powder in olive oil, stirring constantly to prevent burning. Add the chicken broth and bring to a boil. Dissolve the garlic and cornstarch in the water. Stir the water mixture into the broth mixture, stirring constantly to prevent lumps. Add tomato sauce. Serve immediately, refrigerate, or freeze.

Spaghetti Sauce Mix

Small Batch		Large Batch
1 t.	basil	¼ c.
1 t.	oregano	¼ c.
½ t.	marjoram	2 T.
1 t.	sugar	¼ c.
½ t.	salt	2 T.
dash	black pepper	1 t..
2 t.	parsley	½ c.
2 t.	onion powder	½ c.
¾ t.	garlic powder	3 T

Combine all ingredients and put into container with tight-fitting lid. Store at room temperature or in refrigerator for up to one year. Serving size is approximately 3 tablespoons.

Spaghetti Sauce

- 6 oz. tomato paste
- 28 oz. tomatoes
- ½ c. green peppers (optional)
- ⅓ c. water
- 2–3 T. spaghetti sauce mix

Combine all ingredients in a saucepan. Cook about 15 minutes on medium heat. Serve immediately, refrigerate, or freeze.

Creole Seafood Seasoning

   2 T. salt
   2 T. paprika
   1 T. garlic powder
   1 T. onion powder
   1 T. black pepper
1 ½ t. cayenne pepper
1 ½ t. dried thyme
1 ½ t. dried oregano

Combine all ingredients and put into container with tight-fitting lid. Store at room temperature or in refrigerator for up to one year.

Refrigerator Pickles

   1 gal. cucumbers, sliced
   2 large onions, sliced
   1 quart vinegar
   3 c. white sugar
   ¼ c. canning salt (or less)
   1 t. mustard seed
   1 t. celery seed
   1 t. turmeric

Mix cucumbers and onions in a large bowl. Heat vinegar, sugar, and spices to a boil. Let simmer 5 minutes. Pour liquid mixture over cucumbers. When cool, put cucumbers in jars, covering with liquid. Put in refrigerator. In 7 days, they are ready to serve.

Fermented Pickles

   2 cucumbers, sliced or chunked
   1 T. fresh dill or 1 t. dill weed
   ½ t. sea salt
   ½ t. mustard seed
   2 t. whey (for dairy-free, use coconut kefir)
   ½ c. filtered water

Slice cucumbers and pack tightly in 3 pint size mason jars, leaving at least 1–1 ½ inch headspace. Combine the remaining ingredients and pour over cucumbers. Pack the top of the jar with fresh grape leaves to help make the cucumbers more crunchy and to keep the cucumbers under the brine. Be sure the cucumbers remain under the brine so they do not mold. Cover tightly and let stand at room temperature (72 degrees) for about three days. Refrigerate.

I based this recipe on a recipe I found in several books and different places on the internet crediting Sally Fallon, author of Nourishing Traditions, *as the source.*

Fruit Jam

   3 c. fruit (blueberries, raspberries, peaches, apricots, strawberries, or other fruit; peaches and apricots must be peeled and diced)
   2 T. lemon juice
   ½ c. honey
   2 t. gelatin
   3 T. cold water

Sprinkle gelatin in water in saucepan, then set aside for 5 minutes. Add remaining ingredients, then warm over low heat until gelatin is dissolved. Bring to a boil Reduce heat and simmer 10 minutes. Pour into clean, small jars and let cool. Refrigerate or freeze jam.

Pineapple-Kiwi Jam

16 kiwi

7 T. pineapple juice, separated

½ c. sugar

2 t. gelatin

Sprinkle gelatin in 3 T. pineapple juice in saucepan, then set aside for 5 minutes. Cut kiwi in half; scoop out the fruit and place in a separate bowl. Mash the kiwi with a fork or potato masher and add 2 T. pineapple juice. In another bowl, mix sugar and 2 T. pineapple juice until sugar is dissolved. Add kiwi and sugar mixture to gelatin mixture; warm over low heat until gelatin is dissolved. Bring to a boil. Reduce heat and simmer 10 minutes. Pour into clean, small jars and let cool. Refrigerate or freeze jam.

No-Cook Freezer Jam

2 c. prepared fruit (crushed berries or other finely chopped fruit)

1 c. sugar

1 envelope SureJell No-Cook Jam Pectin

½ c. hot water

Mix fruit and sugar in large bowl. Let stand 15 minutes, stirring occasionally. In another bowl, gradually add jam pectin to hot water, stirring constantly. Add to fruit mixture and stir 3 minutes. Pour into clean plastic or glass containers to within 1/2 inch from the top. Seal the jar with a tight-fitting lid. Refrigerate up to 3 weeks or freeze up to 1 year. Thaw in refrigerator. Makes 3 cups of jam.

Perfect recipe for children. My kids LOVE making the jam. I use frozen raspberries, thawed for the fruit. Fresh strawberries work well also. Double this recipe for jam that will last for months.

Apple Pie Freezer Jam

    4 c. chopped, peeled, cored apples (about 5 medium)
    4 c. chopped, peeled, cored pears (about 5 medium)
    ¼ c. water
    1 c. sugar
    ½ c. brown sugar
    ¼ t. cinnamon
    ¼ t. nutmeg
    ¼ t. allspice
    1 package freezer jam pectin

Combine apples, pears, and water in a saucepot. Cover and simmer 5 minutes. Lightly crush fruit. Combine 4 cups cooked fruit, sugars, and spices in a medium bowl. Let stand 15 minutes. Gradually stir freezer jam pectin into fruit mixture. Stir 3 minutes; let stand 5 minutes. Ladle jam into can-or-freeze jars, leaving 1/2 inch headspace. Seal with tight-fitting lid. Label and freeze.

This is a bit time consuming to make, but my kids LOVE it! Pears can be substituted for the apples if apples are not tolerated.

Dried Fruit Spread

    1 c. dried apricots
    1 c. apple juice concentrate

Combine apricots and apple juice concentrate in a saucepan and simmer, uncovered, until the fruit is soft, about 10 minutes. Puree in a blender or food processor until smooth. Use as a spread on bread, pancakes, or waffles, or mix it with plain yogurt.

Mock Cheese

- 1 ½ c. water
- 5 T. unflavored gelatin
- 3/4 c. cashew pieces or tahini
- 1 ¼ t. salt
- 2 t. onion powder
- ¼ t. garlic powder
- ¼ c. pimentos
- 2 ½ T. lemon juice

Combine cashews or tahini with salt, onion powder, garlic powder, pimentos, and lemon juice in a blender or food processor. Boil the water in a small saucepan. Add the gelatin to the water and stir for 1 minute, then add to the other ingredients. Blend for 1–2 minutes, stirring if necessary. Pour into a greased 8" x 8" pan.

This recipe can be frozen. I usually grate the "cheese" before freezing for use in recipes later. This is the only mock cheese recipe I can find. I am not sure of the origin of this recipe, as it appeared in several cookbooks as well as in several places on the internet with no credit given to the author.

Ghee

Place one pound of unsalted organic butter in a heavy saucepan or double boiler. Melt the butter over low heat until completely melted. Continue to cook over low heat until the milk solids on the bottom of the pan turn light brown and the foam at the surface of the butter has nearly evaporated. Be sure to remove the pan from the heat when the milk solids turn golden brown so the ghee will not burn. The butter will then be separated into two parts. The top layer is a translucent liquid called ghee, and the bottom layer contains milk solids. Pour the ghee through a strainer lined with a damp cheesecloth into a heat-proof container. Discard the milk solids or save them for a different recipe. Store ghee covered in a jar for up to 6 months or in the refrigerator for up to one year. Total cooking time is about 30 minutes.

Honey Butter

1 c. butter or dairy-free margarine
½ c. honey

Soften the butter. Mix or blend with honey and store in refrigerator.

Honey Nut Butter

½ c. honey
1 c. nut butter or peanut butter

Combine ingredients in a mixer. Refrigerate or freeze.

Prune Butter/Butter Alternative

- 1 cup pitted prunes
- ½ c. apple juice
- 1 T. orange juice
- ¼ t. vanilla (optional)

Combine ingredients in saucepan. Simmer over low heat for about 1/2 hour, stirring frequently. Cool. Puree in processor until smooth. If too thick, add a little more apple or orange juice. Keep refrigerated in an airtight jar.

This may be used in equal exchange with butter or oil in baked goods. Substitute up to 3/4 of the butter or oil called for in the recipe with prune butter. It works well in brownies and other recipes with cocoa powder, dark muffins, cakes, and cookies. It also tastes great on crackers or on a sandwich with a nut butter. This is based on a recipe from Super Baby Food by Ruth Yaron.

Dairy-Free Sweetened Condensed Milk

- ⅔ c. sugar
- ⅔ c. canned coconut milk
- 3 T. butter, ghee, or allergy-free margarine

On low heat, bring coconut milk to a boil. Remove from heat. Combine milk and sugar, in a blender. Add butter and blend well. Scrape down the sides if needed.

This can be refrigerated for up to 3 weeks or frozen for up to 1 year.

*DariFree powdered milk combined with 2/3 c. of boiling water can be used instead of the canned coconut milk.

Dairy-Free Evaporated Milk

1 c. powdered dairy-free milk*
¾ c. hot water

Combine ingredients in a blender or food processor.

* *DariFree powdered milk works well in this recipe.*

Note: In addition to this recipe, canned coconut milk can also be substituted equally for evaporated milk in recipes.

Strawberry Sauce

1 pint fresh strawberries or raspberries, or 2 c. frozen, thawed
2 T. powdered sugar (optional)
1 T. strawberry preserves

Puree berries in food processor. Blend in the sugar and preserves. Pour sauce into a small saucepan and heat through to blend flavors. Serve warmed, at room temperature, or chilled.

Great for ice cream, pancakes, smoothies, and more.

Brown Sugar Syrup

1 c. brown sugar, packed
½ c. water
½ t. vanilla (optional)
½ t. butter, ghee, or allergy-free margarine (optional)

Combine sugar and water; bring to a boil. Boil for 2 minutes. Remove from heat and stir in vanilla and butter if desired. Serve hot. This can be refrigerated.

We use this for pancakes and waffles and also as a flavoring for plain yogurt. I do not usually add the vanilla or butter. This is high in sugar and should only be used occasionally. Dip pancakes and waffles in the syrup instead of pouring the syrup on top, to reduce consumption of the syrup.

Salad and Soup

Broccoli with Vinaigrette

>   1 lb. broccoli
>   1 t. paprika
>   1 T. mustard
>   1 t. salt
> dash of ground pepper
>   1 T. sugar
>   ¼ c. apple cider vinegar
>   ¼ c. olive oil
>   1 T. chopped olives
>   1 t. grated onion

Steam the broccoli until tender; set aside. Mix the remaining ingredients and heat until the mixture is hot, stirring constantly. Serve hot over the steamed broccoli. Serves 4.

Italian Pasta Salad

>   8 oz. allergy-free pasta, cooked and drained
>   1 cucumber, chopped
>   1 onion, chopped, or 1 bunch of green onions
>   2 stalks of celery, chopped
> 2–3 tomatoes, chopped
>   1 green pepper, chopped
>   allergy-free Italian dressing (p. 101)

Toss ingredients together. Top with Italian dressing about 1 hour before serving. Note: if you add the dressing too early, it will be absorbed into the noodles.

House Salad

1 red onion, diced
2 medium tomatoes, diced
1 cucumber, diced
1 green pepper, diced
1 head of green or red leaf lettuce

Combine all ingredients in a bowl until well mixed. Serve with your favorite dressing.

Vegetable Slaw with Apricot Dressing

Slaw Ingredients:

apples, julienned
celery, julienned
red cabbage, shredded
romaine lettuce, shredded
apricot dressing (recipe below)

Dressing Ingredients:

½ c. apricot preserves, pureed
¼ c. apple cider vinegar
¼–½ c. light olive oil, or grape seed oil
½ t. salt
Pepper to taste

Combine apples, celery, cabbage, and lettuce in a bowl. Set aside. In a small bowl, whisk together the preserves, salt, pepper, and vinegar. Drizzle in the oil while continuing to whisk. (This can also be done in a food processor or blender.) Pour over vegetable mixture and serve immediately. Refrigerate leftovers.

Black Bean Quinoa Salad

    5 T. olive oil
    ½ c. quinoa, rinsed in cold water
    1 c. chicken or vegetable broth
    ¼ t. cumin
    ¼ t. salt
    2 T. lime juice
    ⅛ t. pepper
    1 c. cooked black beans
    1 c. corn
    1 large tomato, diced
    2 green onions, finely chopped
    3 T. cilantro, finely chopped
    2 T. fresh parsley
    2 c. mixed salad greens

Heat 1 tablespoon of oil over medium heat. Add quinoa and stir until toasted (5 minutes), then stir in broth, cumin, and salt. Heat to boiling. Reduce heat to low; cover and simmer until liquid is absorbed (15 minutes). Remove from heat and let stand 5 minutes. Let cool to room temperature. Whisk 4 T. oil, lime, and pepper together. Add beans, corn, tomato, pepper, onions, cilantro, parsley and quinoa to oil mixture. Serve over greens at room temperature or cooled.

Hard-Boiled Eggs

Place eggs in a saucepan filled with water covering the eggs by two inches. Bring the water to a boil; boil for 2 minutes. Cover the pan and remove from heat; let stand for 13 minutes. Remove the eggs from the pan and run under cool water. Peel the eggs. Use immediately or refrigerate until needed. The eggs can be peeled after refrigeration if desired.

Egg Salad

  12 hard-boiled eggs

   3 T. allergy-free mayonnaise *

Peel hard-boiled eggs and place in a bowl. Add mayonnaise and combine until well mixed. Serve warm immediately if eggs were freshly boiled, or refrigerate until ready to serve. Serve on bread, crackers, tortillas, or plain.

A food processor may be used to combine the ingredients well. You can also put plastic baggies on your hands and use your hands to mash the eggs until they are very smooth. This makes the best consistency and is very fast.

*Ranch dressing can be substituted for the mayonnaise.

Mock Jell-O™

  1 c. juice, boiling

  1 c. juice, cold

  1 T. unflavored gelatin

Boil 1 cup of juice. Add gelatin to 1 cup of cold juice. Add boiling juice to cold juice. Stir for 2 minutes. Refrigerate until set, 3–4 hours.

This equals 1 small box of Jell-O from the store. Grape juice works well but stains easily. Orange and apple juices don't work well alone. Try juice combinations such as apple-cherry, apple-cranberry, raspberry, and so on. I have found wonderful combinations from the frozen concentrate section in the grocery store. The Mock Jell-O is faster and healthier than the packaged version you can buy at the store.

Grandma Ruth's Raspberry Salad

   2 c. apple-raspberry juice, boiling

   2 c. apple-raspberry juice, cold

   2 T. unflavored gelatin

   8 oz. frozen raspberries

   2 c. applesauce

Add gelatin to 2 cups of cold juice. Add boiling juice to cold juice. Stir for 2 minutes. Add raspberries and applesauce. Refrigerate until set, 3–4 hours.

My great-grandmother was a professional caterer in southeast Iowa. This dish was a favorite of clients and also a family favorite.

Dairy-Free Coconut Yogurt

   4 c. canned coconut milk

   2 T. agave nectar or honey

   ¼ t. dairy-free yogurt starter*

In a saucepan, combine coconut milk and agave nectar. Heat milk on low heat to 180 degrees, stirring occasionally to prevent sticking. Cool milk to 110–115 degrees. Add yogurt starter to a glass container that is large enough to hold the milk. Once the milk is cooled, add about 2 teaspoons to the yogurt starter to make a paste. Slowly add the remainder of the milk, ½ cup at a time and stirring. Add a lid to the container. Place the container in a warm, insulated place, about 100 degrees, for 6–12 hours. Refrigerate yogurt for up to 5 days or freeze in ice cube trays for up to 3 months. Serve with fresh berries and agave nectar or honey.

*More or less yogurt starter may be used, depending on the brand. Some brands require 1–2 teaspoons per quart of milk. Be sure the starter is dairy-free. I use GI Pro Starter yogurt starter. A firm, edible layer will form over the coconut yogurt.

Dairy-Free Yogurt

    1 c. milk alternative (rice, almond, soy)

¼–½ c. tapioca starch

    ¼ t. dairy-free yogurt starter*

In a saucepan, heat milk alternative on low heat to about 140 degrees, stirring occasionally to prevent sticking. Remove about ½ cup of milk alternative to a mixing bowl while continuing to heat the remainder milk alternative. Whisk the tapioca starch into the ½ cup of separated milk alternative. Slowly whisk the tapioca-milk mix to the saucepan; continue heating until the mixture reaches 180 degrees, stirring frequently. Cool milk mixture to 110–115 degrees. Add yogurt starter to a large glass container. Once the milk is cooled, add about 2 teaspoons of milk mixture to the yogurt starter to make a paste. Slowly add the remainder of the milk, ½ cup at a time, stirring. Place lid on the container. Place the container in a warm, insulated place, about 100 degrees, for 10–24 hours. Refrigerate yogurt for up to 5 days or freeze in ice cube trays for up to 3 months. Serve with fresh berries and agave nectar or honey.

More or less yogurt starter may be used, depending on the brand. Some brands require 1-2 teaspoons per quart of milk. Be sure the starter is dairy-free. I use GI Pro Starter yogurt starter.

Soups

Dairy-Free Cream Soup Substitute #1

2 c. powdered dairy-free milk (we use DariFree)
¾ c. cornstarch or arrowroot powder
2 T. onion flakes
½ t. pepper
1 t. basil
1 t. thyme
2 t. salt

Mix all ingredients well and store in airtight container.

To make sauce: Combine 1/3 cup of mix to 1 1/4 cups of hot broth (chicken, turkey, or beef). Whisk until smooth. Stir often until thickened. This mixture will thicken as it cools.

Combine the ingredients except broth at a more convenient time. When ready to cook, simply add water. You may also mix up several batches at once and store in airtight container until ready to use.

Dairy-Free Cream Soup Substitute #2 (Single Serving)

2 T. powdered dairy-free milk (we use DariFree)
1 T. cornstarch or arrowroot powder
¼ t. onion flakes
dash pepper
dash basil
dash thyme
dash salt

Mix all ingredients well and store in airtight container.

To make sauce: Combine ingredients with 3/4 cup of hot chicken broth. Whisk until smooth. Stir often until thickened. This mixture will thicken as it cools.

Dairy-Free Cream Soup Substitute #3 (Single Serving)

½ c. coconut milk, canned or liquid

½ c. chicken broth

2 t. cornstarch or arrowroot powder

¼ t. onion flakes

dash pepper, basil, thyme and salt

To make sauce: Heat chicken broth with coconut milk until nearly boiling. Add the remainder of the ingredients. Whisk until smooth. Stir often until thickened. This mixture will thicken as it cools.

Old-Fashioned Bean Soup

1 lb. dry navy beans (either soak overnight or bring to a boil and then let soak 1 hour after removing from heat)

7 c. water

½–1 lb. ham

1 medium onion, chopped

½ c. chopped celery leaves

1 t. salt

¼ t. pepper

⅛ t. ginger

Put all ingredients in crockpot. Cover and cook on high for 2 hours. Turn to low and cook 8–10 hours.

Chicken Soup

3 ½ c. chicken broth

1 medium carrot, sliced or diced

1 stalk of celery, sliced or diced

½ c. rice or quinoa

1 c. cubed cooked turkey or chicken

dash ground black pepper

Mix broth, pepper, carrot, and celery in a saucepan. Heat to a boil. Stir in rice or quinoa and chicken. Cook over medium heat 10 minutes or until rice or quinoa is done. *(Leftover rice or quinoa can be used in this recipe.)*

This is adapted from a Swanson brand recipe.

Vegetarian Chili

4–6 scallions, chopped

2 T. olive oil

2 cloves garlic

4 c. or 28 oz. cooked beans (black, red kidney, Great Northern, and so on)

1 t. salt

1 t. allergy-free Worcestershire sauce

1 T. chili powder

6 tomatoes, fresh or frozen, or 2 (26 oz.) cans crushed tomatoes

Sauté onion in oil until transparent. Add minced garlic; cook 1 minute. Add remaining ingredients; heat gently to simmer. Reduce heat and simmer several hours to thicken. Serve plain or over elbow macaroni.

Tortilla Soup

2 boneless chicken breasts

½ t. olive oil

1 c. chopped onion

1 T. lime juice

½ t. minced garlic

½ t. chili powder

¼ t. cumin

3 c. chicken broth

1 c. salsa

1 c. frozen corn (optional)

tortilla chips

Cut chicken into bite-size pieces. Heat oil in frying pan. Add chicken, onion, lime, garlic, chili powder, and cumin. Stir until chicken is cooked. Add broth, salsa, and corn. Cover and bring to boil. Reduce heat and continue to boil for 8–10 minutes. Place small amount of crushed tortilla chips at the bottom of serving bowl. Add soup. Top with cheese or cheese alternative if desired.

To save time, use leftover chicken and then combine all ingredients except chips in a pan and bring to a boil for 8–10 minutes.

Kevin's Chili

    ½ lb. lean ground beef
    1 onion, chopped
    5 cloves garlic
   14 oz. crushed tomatoes, or 2 c. freshly chopped
   14 oz. or 2 c. cooked kidney beans
    1 T. chili powder
    3 dashes of Tabasco (omit if sensitive to vinegar)
    1 t. oregano
    1 t. basil
    1 t. black pepper

Brown beef and drain. Combine all ingredients in a large stockpot. Bring to a medium boil for 30 minutes. Reduce heat and cover. Simmer for a minimum of 1 hour, preferably all day. Add water if necessary. Serve plain or over elbow macaroni. Serves 4–6.

Red Pepper Soup

    2 T. olive oil
    ½ c. onion, chopped
  3–4 red peppers (may be roasted), diced
    2 c. potatoes, raw, peeled and cubed*
  5 ½ c. chicken or vegetable stock
      salt and pepper to taste

In a small stockpot, heat the oil over medium heat. Add the peppers and onion; sauté, stirring about 3 minutes. Add the potatoes, pepper, and stock. Bring the mixture to a boil. Lower heat to a simmer; cover and cook until the potatoes (or rice) are very tender. Add salt and pepper to taste. Puree the soup and serve.

*May substitute 1 cup of uncooked rice.

Use a hand blender to puree the soup in the pot to save time and dishes. Canned roasted red peppers may be used to save time, but nutrients may be lost and it will cost more money.

Vegetable Beef Soup

2 lbs. beef stew meat (optional)
3 c. tomato juice
3 c. beef broth
3 c. water
⅓ c. chopped onion
2 t. salt
2 t. allergy-free Worcestershire sauce (optional)
¼ t. chili powder
3 tomatoes, diced
2 c. diced potatoes (optional)
3 c. mixed vegetables

If using meat, brown beef in small amount of oil in large pot. Add vegetable juice, beef broth, water, and onion. Bring to a boil. Mix in remaining ingredients. Season with salt and pepper. Simmer 3–4 hours. This soup can be frozen.

I usually don't add the meat, tomatoes, or potatoes. A quick way to add potatoes could be using diced frozen potatoes such as Mr. Dell's or other brands without additives or preservatives. If adding potatoes, salt may need to be increased. This soup is fine to eat after one hour of cooking but is not as thick.

Breads and Baked Goods

GLUTEN-FREE BREAD FOR THE MACHINE

	flour mix	salt	xanthan gum	vinegar (optiona
Quickest Bread	3 ⅛ c. all-purpose gluten-free baking flour from package	2 t.	3 t.	¾ t.
Rice Bread	1 ⅛ c. brown rice flour 1 c. cornstarch 1 c. tapioca flour	2 t.	3 t.	¾ t.
Bean Bread #1	1 ⅛ c. garbanzo bean flour 1 c. cornstarch 1 c. tapioca flour	2 t.	3 t.	¾ t.
Bean Bread #2	3/4 c. garbanzo bean flour ⅓ c. sorghum flour 1 c. cornstarch 1 c. tapioca flour	2 t.	3 t.	¾ t.
Bean and Rice Bread	½ c. brown rice flour ½ c. garbanzo bean flour 1 c. cornstarch 1 c. tapioca flour	2 t.	3 t.	¾ t.
Sorghum Bread	1 ½ c. sorghum flour ¾ c. tapioca flour ¾ c. cornstarch	2 t.	3 t.	¾ t.
Oatmeal-Applesauce Bread	any of the above flour mixes	2 t.	3 t.	¾ t.
Carrot Bread	any of the above flour mixes	1 t.	2 t.	¾ t.

rown sugar	eggs	oil	other ingredients	water	dry yeast
2 T.	3	3 T.		1 ⅛ c. warm water	2 t. or 1 packet
2 T.	3	3 T.		1 ⅛ c. warm water	2 t. or 1 packet
2 T.	3	3 T.		1 ⅛ c. warm water	2 t. or 1 packet
2 T.	3	3 T.		1 ⅛ c. warm water	2 t. or 1 packet
2 T.	3	3 T.		1 ⅛ c. warm water	2 t. or 1 packet
2 T.	3	3 T.		1 ⅛ c. warm water	2 t. or 1 packet
	3	2 T.	⅓ c. oatmeal ⅓ c. applesauce 1 t. cinnamon 1 T. molasses	1 ¼ c. warm water	2 t. or 1 packet
3 T.	2	4 T.	1 c. grated carrots ¾ t. cinnamon 4 T. powdered milk or milk substitute	1 ⅛ c. warm water	2 t. or 1 packet

	flour mix	salt	xanthan gum	vinegar (optional)
Lemon-Poppy Seed Bread	any of the above flour mixes	2 t.	3 t.	¾ t.
Raisin Bread	any of the above flour mixes	2 t.	3 t.	¾ t.
Cranberry Bread	any of the above flour mixes	2 t.	3 t.	¾ t.
Cranberry-Orange Bread	any of the above flour mixes	2 t.	3 t.	¾ t.
Apricot Bread	any of the above flour mixes	2 t.	3 t.	¾ t.
Egg-Free Bread	any of the above flour mixes	2 t.	3 t.	¾ t.
Herb Bread	any of the above flour mixes	2 t.	3 t.	¾ t.
Potato Bread	any of the above flour mixes	2 t.	3 t.	¾ t.
Zucchini Bread	any of the above flour mixes	2 t.	3 t.	¾ t.
Millet Bread	any of the above flour mixes	2 t.	3 t.	¾ t.

rown sugar	eggs	oil	other ingredients		water	dry yeast
2 T.	3	3 T.	2 t. lemon zest 3 t. poppy seeds		1 ⅛ c. warm water	2 t. or 1 packet
2 T.	3	3 T.	¼ c. raisins 1 t. cinnamon		1 ⅛ c. warm water	2 t. or 1 packet
4 T.	3	3 T.	¼ c. dried cranberries ¼ c. chopped nuts 1 ½ t. dried orange peel 1/2 c. cranberry juice		3/4 c. warm water	2 t. or 1 packet
4 T.	3	3 T.	¼ c. dried cranberries ¼ c. chopped nuts 1 ½ t. dried orange peel ½ c. cranberry juice		½ c. warm water	2 t. or 1 packet
4 T.	3	3 T.	⅓ c. almond meal ⅓ c. dried apricots, chopped ¾ c. apricot nectar		¾ c. warm water	2 t. or 1 packet
2 T.		3 T.	3 T. chia seeds combined with 9 T. water		1 ⅛ c. warm water	2 t. or 1 packet
2 T.	3	3 T.	3 T. dried parsley flakes 2 T. dill 2 T. caraway seeds		1 ¼ c. warm water	2 t. or 1 packet
2 T.	3	3 T.	¼ c. instant mashed potato flakes		1 ¼ c. warm water	2 t. or 1 packet
2 T.	3		¼ c. grated zucchini 1 ½ t. cinnamon 1 t. ground cloves ⅓ c. nuts		1 c. warm water	2 t. or 1 packet
	3	3 T.	⅓ c. millet flour ¼ c. rice bran 2 T. molasses		½ c. warm water	2 t. or 1 packet

	flour mix	salt	xanthan gum	vinegar (optiona
Apple-Raisin Bread	any of the above flour mixes	2 t.	3 t.	¾ t.
Sweet Potato Bread	any of the above flour mixes	2 t.	3 t.	¾ t.
Quinoa Bread	any of the above flour mixes	2 t.	3 t.	¾ t.
Ancient Grain Bread	any of the above flour mixes	2 t.	3 t.	¾ t.

Note: In all of the above recipes, the salt can be reduced to 1 or 1½ teaspoons. The brown sugar can be equally replaced with molasses, blackstrap molasses, organic sugar, honey, or agave nectar. The eggs can all be substituted with an egg substitute, but the end result may not be the same.

rown sugar	eggs	oil	other ingredients	water	dry yeast
1 T.	3	3 T.	⅓ c. applesauce 1 t. cinnamon ⅓ c. raisins	1 c. warm water	2 t. or 1 packet
½ c.	3	3 T.	⅓ c. mashed sweet potato 1 ½ c. cranberries	1 ⅛ c. warm water	2 t. or 1 packet
3 T.	3	4 T.	3 T. quinoa flour or flakes	1 ½ c. warm water	2 t. or 1 packet
3 T.	3	4 T.	2 T. quinoa flour or flakes 2 T. amaranth flour	1 ½ c. warm water	2 t. or 1 packet

Gluten-Free Bread for Machine

3 ⅛ c. gluten-free flour mix

1 ½ t. salt

3 ½ t. xanthan gum

2 T. brown sugar or blackstrap molasses

¼ t. ascorbic acid or vinegar (optional)

3 eggs, beaten

1 ⅛ c. warm water

3 T. oil

2 ¼ t. or 1 packet yeast

Place ingredients in bread machine according to manufacturer's directions. Press start button. Or, dissolve yeast in warm water for 5 minutes. Combine flour, salt, xanthan gum, and brown sugar in a small bowl. Combine eggs, water with dissolved yeast, and oil in bread machine bucket. Add dry ingredients. Set to "light" cycle. Press start.

This is the best machine bread yet! This is as close as I could come to "regular" bread. The blackstrap molasses gives the bread extra nutrient content but gives the bread a bit of a different flavor. My son likes it with either the brown sugar or the molasses. This bread freezes well.

Egg-Free Bean Bread for Machine

 1 c. tapioca starch

 1 c. potato starch or cornstarch

 ¾ c. garbanzo bean flour or garfava flour

 ⅓ c. sorghum flour

 3 t. xanthan gum

 3 T. oil

 2 T. brown sugar

1 ½ t. salt

 3 T. flax meal combined with 9 T. warm water

1⅛ c. water or milk alternative

2 ¼ t. or 1 packet yeast dissolved in the water or milk

Place ingredients in bread machine according to manufacturer's directions. Press start button. Or, dissolve yeast in warm water for 5 minutes. Combine flour, salt, xanthan gum, and brown sugar in a small bowl. Combine flax meal mixture, water or milk with dissolved yeast, and oil in bread machine bucket. Add dry ingredients. Set to "light" cycle. Press start. This bread freezes well.

Egg-Free Rice Bread for Machine

1 c. tapioca starch

1 c. potato starch or cornstarch

1 c. brown rice flour

3 t. xanthan gum

3 T. oil

3 T. brown sugar

1 ½ t. salt

3 T. flax meal or ground chia seed combined with 9 T. warm water

1 ⅛ c. water or milk alternative

2 ¼ t. or 1 packet yeast, dissolved in the water or milk

Place ingredients in bread machine according to manufacturer's directions. Press start button. Or, dissolve yeast in warm water for 5 minutes. Combine flour, salt, xanthan gum, and brown sugar in a small bowl. Combine flax meal mixture, water or milk with dissolved yeast, and oil in bread machine bucket. Add dry ingredients. Set to "light" cycle. Press start. This bread freezes well.

Yeast- and Egg-Free Quinoa Bread

1¼ c. brown rice flour

1 c. tapioca starch

¾ c. potato starch or cornstarch

1 c. garbanzo bean flour or garfava flour

¼ c. flax meal

2 t. xanthan gum

2 T. baking powder

¾ t. salt

¼ c. oil

1 ½ c. apple cider, apple juice, or pear juice

½ c. unsweetened applesauce, pearsauce, or pureed sweet potato

1 T. honey

1 T. apple cider vinegar (optional)

½ c. cooked whole-grain quinoa or millet

Preheat oven to 400 degrees. Combine dry ingredients in a medium bowl. Fold in the cooked quinoa to the dry ingredients. In a separate bowl, combine applesauce, juice, honey, cider vinegar, and oil with a mixer. Add the dry ingredients to the wet ingredients and blend on medium speed until just combined. Do not over mix. Place batter in a greased loaf pan dusted with cornmeal or rice flour. Cover with foil and bake for 40 minutes. Remove foil and bake, uncovered, for 15 more minutes. If needed, recover the bread and cook until the internal temperature reaches 200 degrees, approximately 15 more minutes. This bread freezes well.

For increased nutrients, subtract ¼ c. brown rice flour and ¼ c. bean flour and add ¼ c. teff and ¼ c. millet. Pearsauce is often sold as baby food and can be found in the baby food aisle at most stores. Pearsauce can also be made by following the Crockpot Applesauce recipe in this book using pears instead of apples. This recipe is adapted from Living Without magazine, found at wwwlivingwithout.com. This is our favorite egg-free bread.

Yeast-Free Rice Bread

  1 c. tapioca starch
  1 c. corn starch
  2 c. brown rice flour
  2 t. xanthan gum
  2 T. brown sugar
  1 t. baking soda
  4 t. baking powder
  1 t. salt
  3 eggs*
  6 T. oil
  1 ½ c. rice milk or other milk alternative

Combine dry ingredients in a medium bowl. Combine wet ingredients with a mixer. Add the dry ingredients to the wet ingredients and blend on low until well blended. Batter will be slightly runny. Add ¼–½ c. of water if the batter is solid. Place batter in 2 greased loaf pans and bake at 350 degrees for 40 minutes. This bread freezes well.

*The eggs can be replaced with an egg substitute, but the bread does not rise as well with the egg substitute.

This recipe is based on Basic Yeast-Free Rice Bread from The Gluten-Free Gourmet Bakes Bread by Bette Hagman. This book is excellent for bread recipes!

Yeast- and Egg-Free Bean Bread

   1 c. tapioca starch

   1 c. potato or corn starch

   ⅔ c. garbanzo bean flour or garfava flour

   ⅓ c. sorghum flour

   2 t. xanthan gum

   2 T. brown sugar

   1 t. baking soda

   4 t. baking powder

4 ½ T. oil

   1 t. salt

   3 T. flax meal combined with 9 T. warm water*

1 ½ c. milk or milk alternative

Combine dry ingredients in a medium bowl. Combine wet ingredients with a mixer. Add the dry ingredients to the wet ingredients and blend on low until well blended. Batter will be slightly runny. Add ¼–½ c. of water if the batter is too thick. Place batter in 2 greased loaf pans and bake at 350 degrees for 40 minutes. This bread freezes well.

*Any egg substitute can be used to equal 3 eggs.

Rice Bread

    2 ½ c. warm water
      1 T. yeast
      1 T. oil
      ½ t. salt
      ½ c. sunflower seeds
      ¼ c. gluten-free rolled oats
      ¼ c. garbanzo bean flour
      2 c. rice flour
      ½ c. millet flour

Combine yeast and water in a bowl. Set aside. Combine dry ingredients
in a medium bowl. Add the dry ingredients to the wet ingredients and
blend on low until well blended. Batter will be runny. Place batter in
2 greased loaf pans and let rise uncovered for 20–30 minutes. Bake at
350 degrees for 60 minutes. Cool 3–5 minutes, then remove bread from
the pan to cool. Handle the batter gently at all times or the bread may
collapse. This bread freezes well.

Classic Pancakes

      2 eggs, well beaten
      ½ c. milk or milk alternative
      2 T. oil
      ¾ c. gluten-free flour mix
      2 t. baking powder
      ½ t. xanthan gum
      ½ t. salt
      1 t. sugar

Beat together eggs, milk, and oil. Sift together flour, baking powder,
salt, xanthan gum, and sugar in another bowl. Stir into egg mixture
until all ingredients are well blended. Cook on hot griddle. Be sure to
spread the batter to make it thin on the griddle or the middle may not
get cooked evenly.

*Be sure the griddle is hot or the first batch will turn out like crepes instead of
pancakes. I use Bette Hagman's gluten-free Featherlight mix for the pancakes.*

Pumpkin Waffles

- 16 oz. canned pumpkin
- ⅓ c. brown sugar
- ½ c. milk, milk alternative, or water
- ¼ c. melted butter, ghee, or oil
- 2 eggs
- 2 t. baking powder
- ¼ t. salt
- ¼ t. baking powder
- ¼ t. pumpkin pie spice
- 1 c. gluten-free flour mix

In a large bowl, mix pumpkin, sugar, milk, butter, and eggs. In another bowl, combine dry ingredients. Add dry ingredients to wet ingredients and mix. Pour into waffle iron. Cook until browned, 4–6 minutes.

For a variation, try adding 1/2 cup dried cranberries rehydrated in 1/4 cup water.

Bagels

- 2 c. tapioca flour
- 2 c. rice flour
- 4 T. dried milk powder or milk alternative powder
- 3 t. xanthan gum
- 1 ½ t. salt
- 3 T. sugar, divided
- 1 c. warm water
- 2 ½ t. or 1 packet yeast
- 4 T. butter, ghee, or allergy-free margarine
- ½ c. hot water
- 2 eggs

Place all dry ingredients except 1 1/2 teaspoons sugar and yeast in the bowl of a heavy-duty mixer. Stir the dry mixture with a dough hook on low speed. Add the remaining sugar with 1 cup of warm water and yeast; set aside. Add the butter to the 1/2 cup of hot water until the butter is dissolved, then add this mixture to the dry ingredients. Blend the two mixtures. Blend in the eggs, then add the yeast mixture. Beat on high for 4 minutes. Add flour if the dough is too runny; add water if the dough needs thickened.

Divide the dough into 16 equal portions. Roll the portions into balls. Gently poke a hole in the center of each ball of dough and enlarge it to the size of a quarter. (You can also roll the portions into a log and form a circle with the log by pressing the ends together.) Place on a greased baking pan, sprinkle with water, and cover lightly with plastic wrap or a light towel. Letthedoughrise30–60minutes. (I place the dough in the unheated oven with the light on to create a humid environment for rising.)

Bring 1 gallon of water plus 1 teaspoon of sugar to boil, then reduce to a simmer. Place 4–5 bagels at a time in the water and cook for 1 minute, turning once. Drain well. Place the boiled bagels on a greased baking pan. Bake in a 450 degree oven 20–25 minutes, turning them over halfway through baking.

The bagels freeze nicely. I adapted this recipe from Sarah's Bagels in The Gluten-Free Gourmet Bakes Bread by Bette Hagman. It is a great book for gluten-free bread recipes. The bagels do not work well with coconut oil as a substitute for the butter.

My autistic son's first prayer came at Thanksgiving time when he was nearly 5 years old. He said, "Dear God, thank you for making bagels. Amen!" This is one of his favorite recipes.

Pizza Crust

- ⅔ c. brown rice flour
- ½ c. tapioca starch
- ½ t. sugar
- 2 t. xanthan gum
- ½ t. salt
- 1 t. unflavored gelatin
- 1 c. warm water
- 1 t. yeast
- 1 t. olive oil

In medium bowl using regular beaters (not dough hooks), blend the brown rice flour, tapioca starch, sugar, xanthan gum, salt, and gelatin on low speed. Combine warm water, yeast and olive oil in a small bowl. Add warm water and olive oil. Mix all ingredients together. Oil your fingers, then press the dough on a greased 12" pizza pan or baking sheet, or spread the dough out in smaller, individual portions. Bake at 350 degrees for 10 minutes. At this point, the dough and individual portions can be taken out of the oven and then frozen, or remove the dough from the oven and add pizza ingredients such as sauce and toppings. Bake an additional 15–20 minutes or until toppings are well cooked and dough is lightly brown. If the dough was frozen, remove from the freezer and add pizza toppings, then bake at 350 degrees for 20–25 minutes or until dough is lightly brown and toppings are well cooked.

This dough is based on a recipe from Carol Fenster, PhD, author of Special Diet Solutions and other dietary cookbooks. This is our favorite and easiest pizza crust to make.

Savory Pie Crust

¾ c. white rice flour

¼ c. potato starch

½ t. xanthan gum

½ t. salt

1 t. baking powder

⅔ c. butter, ghee, or allergy-free margarine

1 egg

¾ c. water

Preheat oven to 425 degrees. Grease a 10" pie pan or baking dish; set aside. Place all ingredients in a small mixing bowl. Mix on medium speed until just blended, less than 2 minutes. Spread batter in prepared pie pan or dish. Carefully spoon filling into center of batter. Do not stir. Bake for 35 minutes, until crust is golden brown.

This makes a biscuit mix-type crust. Use this for chicken pot pie or other dishes with a thick biscuit crust.

Potato Crust

3 c. grated raw potato

1–2 T. oil

Combine ingredients. Press into 9" pie pan and bake for 15 minutes at 350 degrees until it just starts to brown. Add quiche filling and bake.

If making a quiche, you may need to reduce the eggs to 3 in your recipe because of the thick crust, or use fewer potatoes for a thinner crust.

Rice Crust

3 c. brown rice

2 eggs, beaten

Combine ingredients. Press into 9" pie pan and bake for 15 minutes at 350 degrees until it just starts to brown. Cover with foil to prevent burning. Add quiche or other filling and bake.

Cornmeal Crust

 2 c. water

 ½ t. salt

 1 egg

 1 c. yellow cornmeal

Bring water to boil. Whisk cornmeal in slowly. After the cornmeal is cooked, add egg and salt; mix well. Press into pizza pan or casserole dish. Bake at 400 degrees for 20 to 25 minutes.

Corn Chips

 1 c. warm water

 1 egg yolk

 1 t. salt

 ¾ c. mesa harina, or as needed

 oil for frying

In a mixing bowl, whisk the water, egg yolk, and salt together. Gradually add enough mesa harina to make a soft dough that does not stick to your fingers. In a heavy skillet, preheat oil at least 2 inches deep to 375 degrees. Fit a cookie press or pastry bag with the plate designed to make a flat ribbed shape and fill it with the mesa dough. Press out into the hot oil a few short lengths of dough, enough to cover about half of the pan. Fry the dough, turning once, just until golden brown. Lift the chips from the oil with a slotted spoon and drain on paper towels.

Serve immediately or cool completely and store in an airtight container. To serve chips after storage, place them briefly in a warm oven. They will keep for up to 1 week.

Fruits and Vegetables

Chunky Applesauce

5–12 apples

Peel and cut desired amount of apples into ½ –1-inch chunks. Place the chunks in the slow cooker and add about ½ cup water. Set the cooker on low and cook 4–6 hours, or until apples are soft. Mash with a potato masher to desired consistency.

This recipe may be frozen. Refrigerate uneaten portions. To save time, make a large batch and freeze. To save money, use free or local apples.

Greek Salad

 2 large cucumbers, diced
 2 tomatoes, diced
 2 green peppers, diced
 ¼ c. black olives (optional)
 6 green onions, diced
 ½ c. allergy-free Italian dressing (more or less)
    Feta cheese (optional)

Toss cucumbers, tomatoes, peppers, and olives in a bowl. Add enough Italian dressing to cover vegetables but not have excess dressing. Stir mixture. Top with Feta cheese after serving. This mixture can be used as a topping for lettuce or as a side dish of its own.

Spicy Sweet Potatoes

  3 large sweet potatoes, peeled and in 1" cubes
  2 T. olive oil
  1 T. brown sugar
  ¼ t. chili powder
  ½ t. salt
dash cayenne pepper, or to taste

Toss cubed sweet potatoes and oil in plastic bag or tight container. Add remaining ingredients. Toss to coat. Pour in a 9" x 13" pan. Bake 400 degrees for 40 to 45 minutes or until tender. Stir every 15 minutes. This recipe freezes well.

Spicy Sweet Potato French Fries

  12 large sweet potatoes, peeled
  8 T. olive oil
  4 T. brown sugar
  1 t. chili powder
  2 t. salt
  ¼ t. cayenne pepper, or to taste

Slice potatoes in 1/4" strips. Toss sweet potatoes and oil in plastic bag or tightly sealed container. Mix and add remaining ingredients. Toss to coat. Put on four baking sheets or 9" x 13" pans. Bake at 400 degrees for 40 to 45 minutes or until tender. Stir every 15 minutes. For crispy fries, freeze after cooking and reheat in the oven for 20 to 25 minutes or until crisp. Makes 32 servings. Fries can be frozen.

Sweet Potato Soufflé

  3–4 fresh sweet potatoes (3 cups) cooked & mashed*

  ½ c. sugar

  ½ t. salt

  2 eggs, slightly beaten

  1 c. coconut milk**

t. allergy-free vanilla (optional)

Topping:

  ½ c. allergy-free cereal such as crispy rice, cornflakes,
Rice Crunch Ems or Corn Crunch Ems, etc.

  ¼ c. (or less) brown sugar, packed

  2 T. butter, ghee, or allergy-free margarine

* Butternut squash can be substituted.

**Evaporated milk or dairy-free evaporated milk can be substituted.

Preheat oven to 350 degrees. In a mixing bowl, beat sugar, salt, eggs, coconut milk, and vanilla. Stir in squash (mixture will be thin). Pour into a greased 7" x 11" baking pan. Bake uncovered for 45 minutes or until almost set. Combine topping ingredients; sprinkle over casserole. Return to oven for 5 to 10 minutes or until bubbly. Serves 6–8.

This is a huge hit at holidays, even with non-allergen guests!

Baked Squash

Cut squash in half and remove seeds. Place in baking dish, skin side up, in about 1" water. Bake at 350 degrees for 40 minutes or until tender. Remove from oven and fill each cavity with 1 T. brown sugar if desired. Continue to bake for 10 min.

Ranch Roasted Potatoes

6-8   potatoes, peeled and cut into 1" cubes

1   T. allergy-free ranch mix, purchased, or using recipe on p. 98

¼   c. oil

Combine oil and ranch mix. Place cubed potatoes and oil mix in an air-tight container. Toss to coat and place in a 9" x 13" baking pan. Bake at 450 degrees for 40 to 45 minutes or until tender and golden brown, stirring every 15 minutes. This recipe freezes well.

Garlic & Rosemary Potatoes

2   lbs. red potatoes (4–5 large), unpeeled

2   garlic cloves, pressed

1   T. dried rosemary

¼   t. salt

¼   c. olive oil

Cut potatoes in half and cut each half into 4 wedges about 1" wide. In a bowl, combine potatoes with oil. Press garlic over potatoes and sprinkle with rosemary and salt. Spread potatoes in single layer on baking dish. Bake 10 minutes. Turn potatoes and continue baking 10–15 minutes or until light golden brown and tender.

Scalloped Potatoes

4–5   potatoes, sliced

2   T. butter, ghee, or allergy-free margarine

2   T. cornstarch

1 ¼   c. milk or coconut milk

1 ¼   t. salt

dash of cayenne pepper or chili powder, or to taste

Make white sauce by melting the butter in a pan. Add cornstarch, salt, and then milk or coconut milk. Cook until thick. Pour potatoes in a casserole dish or pan. Pour the sauce over the potatoes and bake at 350 degrees until potatoes are done, about 1 hour.

If you want to get done in a hurry, bring the potatoes to a boil or steam the potatoes for 15 minutes while making the white sauce. Then cook the scalloped potatoes for 20 to 30 minutes.

French Fries

    5 large potatoes
    ¼ c. olive oil
       salt to taste

Cut potatoes in half lengthwise, making the slices about 1/4" thick
or less. Cut each slice into thin strips about 1/4" thick or less to make
French fry sticks. Place the potatoes in a 9" x 13" pan and brush lightly
with oil. Sprinkle with salt (about 1 teaspoon, or to taste). Bake at 350
degrees for an hour or until potatoes are tender and lightly brown. Serve
or freeze.

*For crispy fries, freeze the fries and then re-cook on a baking stone or cookie
sheet. I found my kids eat the fries if they are the same size as fast food fries.
Experiment with size of fries and more or less oil to fit your family's tastes. I
don't peel my potatoes, and I always use organic potatoes or potatoes fresh from
my garden.*

*Make several batches of the French fries at the same time and freeze the
portion you don't eat. I usually make 4 batches at once. Buy a large amount
of potatoes while they are on sale or fresh from the farmers market in the fall.
Make large batches of each recipe above and freeze them. Better yet, grow
them in your garden and make large batches when it is time to harvest.*

Fried Potato Cubes

    4 potatoes, peeled and in 1/4" cubes
    ¼ t. garlic powder
    ¼ t. onion salt
    ¼ c. oil for frying

Heat a medium skillet on high to warm the pan. When the pan is warm,
add oil. Add potatoes and cook on high heat until they begin to brown,
approximately 2 minutes. Add garlic powder and onion salt. Turn heat to
medium and cook until potatoes are cooked through, tender and brown,
approximately 15 minutes. Serve immediately. *Small cubes will cook faster.*

Potato Pancakes

    2 eggs

    1 T. flour or cornstarch

    ½ t. salt

    2 t. minced onion

    2 potatoes, grated

    4 slices bacon, cooked and crumbled (optional)

    1 c. warm applesauce

dash nutmeg

Combine eggs, flour, salt, onion, and potatoes. Spoon 1/4 cup of batter into hot greased griddle at a time; flatten and cook on both sides until lightly browned. Sprinkle with crumbled bacon and spoon warm applesauce over tops.

To save time, you can use uncooked frozen hashbrown potatoes instead of the 2 potatoes. Be sure the potatoes are allergy-free and free of unhealthy oils and preservatives. I like Mr. Dell's brand frozen potatoes.

Iowa Freezer Corn

    20 c. corn

    5 c. water, ice cold

    ½ c. sugar (much less if corn is sweet)

    ¼ c. salt

Combine all ingredients and freeze in desired containers.

Grilled Corn and Veggies

6 cleaned ears of corn
⅓ c. olive oil
2 t. lime juice
salt and pepper to taste
¼ " slices of zucchini, eggplant, or summer squash

Place all ingredients in a large plastic bag. Shake well. Place corn on outdoor grill. Grill corn for about 6 minutes, rotating frequently, until tender-crisp. Brush other vegetables generously with oil and lime juice. Grill until just tender-crisp.

Squash and Pepper Skillet

1 medium onion, thinly sliced
1 T. olive oil
5 medium zucchini, sliced
3 medium yellow summer squash, sliced
1 green or red pepper, julienned
1 garlic clove
salt and pepper to taste

In a skillet, sauté the onion in oil until tender. Add the zucchini, yellow squash, red pepper, and garlic; stir-fry for 12 to 15 minutes or until vegetables are crisp-tender. Season with salt and pepper. Can be served over rice or pasta or served as a side dish.

Roasted Vegetables

potatoes	peppers	asparagus
mushrooms	green beans	onions
other vegetables		

Place vegetables on an ungreased baking sheet. Spray lightly with spray oil or very lightly brush with olive oil. Roast in a 375-degree oven for 10 minutes for most vegetables and 30–40 minutes for potatoes. Sprinkle with herb seasoning if desired. This can be reheated if undercooked in the first roasting.

Oven-Baked Herbed Rice

- 1 c. brown rice
- 2 c. boiling water
- ¼ t. sage
- ¼ t. thyme
- ¼ t. pepper
- ¼ t. parsley
- 1 T. chicken broth
- 2 T. butter, ghee, or allergy-free margarine (optional)
- chopped onions (optional)
- chopped mushrooms (optional)

Pour all ingredients in a 1 1/2-quart casserole dish. Bake at 350 degrees for 45 to 50 minutes.

Spanish Rice #1

- 8 small frozen tomatoes, thawed, with skins removed, or 24 oz. can stewed tomatoes
- 1 green pepper, diced
- 2–4 T. dried onion
- 1–2 t. salt
- 1 t. celery seed
- 2 minced garlic cloves

4–5 c. cooked rice

Combine all ingredients on medium heat until tomatoes break down, approximately 15 minutes. Add to rice. This makes 4–6 meals for our family. Freeze the unused rice in freezer bags or in glass jars.

Simply pull out a freezer bag when you need Spanish rice, and thaw overnight in the refrigerator or in a container of water at room temperature.

Spanish Rice #2

1 c. brown rice (not instant)
olive oil or quality cooking oil
1 (16) oz. can crushed tomatoes or 2 c. tomatoes (seeded and skins removed) or 2 c. frozen tomatoes (skins removed and thawed)
¾ c. chicken broth
1 serving of Spanish rice mix (see below), fresh or dried

If desired, sauté rice in olive oil until lightly browned. Add chicken broth and tomatoes to the pan until broken down and rice is cooked. Add one serving of either fresh or dried Spanish rice mix. This recipe freezes well.

Fresh Spanish Rice Mix

1–2 garlic cloves
4 T. celery, chopped
4 T. green pepper, chopped
2 T. dried onion
dash pepper flakes (optional)
1 t. salt

Combine all ingredients and add to Spanish rice #2. Makes one serving.

Dried Spanish Rice Mix

Small Batch	Large Batch
dash red pepper flakes	4 dashes
1 T. dried celery flakes	¼ c.
2 T. dried green peppers	½ c.
1 T. dried onion	¼ c.
½ t. sea salt	2 t.
⅛ T. garlic powder	1 t.

Combine all ingredients and shake well. The small batch is one serving and equals 1/4 cup.

Cooking Dried Beans

    1 lb. dried beans

    10 c. water

In a strainer, rinse the beans well. Discard any discolored or shriveled beans.

Overnight Soak:

In a large saucepan, cover beans with water. Cover tightly and refrigerate 6–8 hours or overnight. Drain and rinse the beans.

Quick Soak:

In a large saucepan, bring the water to a boil. Add the beans and return to a boil for 2 to 3 minutes. Cover tightly and remove from heat. Set aside at room temperature for one hour. Drain and rinse the beans.

Stovetop Cooking:

Return the beans to the saucepan and cover with water three times the volume of the beans. Bring the water to a boil and simmer gently, uncovered, until the beans are tender, 1–1 ½ hours. Be sure to add more water if the water level is low. The beans are done when they can be mashed with a fork. When the beans are done cooking, drain the water and use the beans immediately or refrigerate for several days. Yield: 5–6 cups.

Crockpot Cooking:

Use the overnight-soak method in the crockpot with the beans and water. Place the beans back into the crockpot after draining. Cover the beans with water (at least 3 inches over the beans). Cover and cook on low for 8 hours or until the beans are tender.

Refried Beans

    1 onion, chopped
    2 T. olive oil
    4 cloves garlic
    4 c. pinto or black beans, cooked
    1 c. water or cooking liquid
       salt to taste

Heat the oil in a skillet over medium heat. Add the onion and sauté
for about 10 minutes, until deep golden brown. Add garlic and cook,
stirring often, for 1 minute. Add beans 1 cup at a time, mashing each
addition of beans to a puree with a potato masher or back of a large
spoon before adding the next cupful. Stir in water. Cook, stirring often,
over medium to low heat until the beans are soupier than to be served.
They will thicken upon sitting. Season with salt. The beans can be
frozen for up to 3 months.

Crockpot Baked Beans

    1 lb. dried beans*
 4 ½ c. water
    ⅓ c. molasses
    ¼ c. brown sugar
    1 onion, chopped
    ¼ lb. bacon, about 8 strips, cooked and sliced
    1 T. dry mustard
    1 t. salt

Combine all ingredients in a crockpot. Cover and cook on low 13–14
hours, stirring occasionally if possible. This recipe can be frozen.

Kidney, black, pinto, or navy beans are good choices for this recipe.

Baked Beans

  1 ½ lb. dried beans, cooked*
    ¼ c. molasses
    ¼ c. brown sugar
    1 onion, chopped
    ¼ lb. bacon, about 8 strips
    1 T. dry mustard
    1 t. salt
  28 oz. tomatoes, crushed

Combine all ingredients. Bake, covered, in a 375-degree oven for 1 hour. This recipe can be frozen.

Kidney, black, pinto, or navy beans are good choices for this recipe.

Grilled Eggplant

  1 eggplant
     olive oil
     lemon juice
     garlic
     sage
     pepper

Slice eggplant into 1/2"-thick round slices. Heavily salt both sides of sliced eggplant and place on a paper towel to dry for 1 hour. Wash off salt. Brush olive oil and lemon juice over surface. Add flavorings. Place on grill until browned on both sides.

Eggplant Parmesan #1

   1 eggplant
  24 oz. allergy-free tomato sauce
  16 oz. shredded mozzarella cheese or cheese alternative

Slice eggplant into 1/2" slices. Boil the eggplant in water until it is mushy but still holds its shape. Grease a 9" x 13" pan. Cover bottom of pan with a light layer of sauce. Lay cooked eggplant evenly over the pan. Pour rest of sauce on top of the eggplant. Top with cheese alternative. Bake at 350 degrees for 20 to 30 minutes or until cheese is bubbly.

Eggplant Parmesan #2

   1 eggplant
 2–3 eggs
   2 c. gluten-free bread crumbs or rice crackers
  24 oz. allergy-free tomato sauce
  16 oz. shredded mozzarella cheese or cheese alternative (optional)
      oil for frying

Slice eggplant into 1/2" slices. Warm a skillet to medium heat. Place the eggs in a small bowl and blend yolks and whites well. Put bread crumbs in another small bowl. Dip the eggplant into the egg mixture and then into the bread crumbs. Add oil to cover the bottom of the skillet. Fry the eggplant until the bottom is browned. Turn over and fry the other side of the eggplant until browned and eggplant is cooked. Place the fried eggplant pieces side-by-side in a greased 9" x 13" pan. Top with tomato sauce and cheese. Bake at 350 degrees until cheese is bubbly, or until heated through if not using cheese, about 20 minutes. Serve as a side dish, over pasta, or on a sandwich.

This takes a little bit of time to make but is a family favorite. I love saving the leftovers to use on sandwiches or on French bread.

Main Dishes

Beans and Rice

    1 onion, diced
    1 green pepper, diced
    1 garlic clove, minced
    1 t. cumin
    2 T. olive oil
    8 oz. tomato sauce
    2 c. canned red, kidney, or black beans, undrained *

In a large skillet, sauté onion, garlic, green pepper, and cumin in oil. Add tomato sauce and beans. Cook on medium heat until beans are cooked through. Serve over cooked rice.

*Dried beans can be used but must be cooked prior to using. Add about 1/4–1/2 cup of liquid with the beans.

Bean Burritos

    5 c. cooked pinto or black beans, mashed
    2 t. salt
  2–4 t. cumin
  ½–1 t. paprika
pinch cayenne pepper
    1 t. onion powder
    1 t. garlic powder
    1 c. cooked chicken or hamburger (optional)
   15 oz. tomato sauce
    ½ c. salsa
    1 small onion
      cheddar cheese or cheese alternative to top (optional)
   12 tortillas

Add salt and spices (and meat, if used) to mashed beans; set aside. In blender or food processor, liquefy tomato sauce, salsa, and onion. Water may be added to this mixture, if needed. To assemble, spread a fair amount of bean mixture down the center of each tortilla, and sprinkle with cheese, if used. Roll tightly and place side by side in a greased 9" x 13" pan. Pour tomato or enchilada sauce over all. Bake at 325 degrees for 20 to 30 minutes. Sprinkle with more cheese and parsley for garnish.

Fajitas

    8 oz. portabella mushrooms, sliced, or 8 oz. of beef or chicken,
      cooked and cut into strips
  ½–1 c. of picante sauce or salsa
    1 green pepper, sliced lengthwise
    1 onion, sliced lengthwise
    2 T. oil
Sauté onions, green peppers, and mushrooms, if using, in oil. Add beef or chicken. Add picante sauce and cook until sauce has thickened on peppers and onions. Serve in tortillas. Garnish with lettuce, cheese, and tomatoes if desired.

Easy Crockpot Fajitas

   1 boneless beef or deer roast
   1 onion, chopped
   2 T. allergy-free taco seasoning mix p. 103

Place roast and onions in crockpot. Sprinkle seasoning over roast. Cook on low 8–10 hours. Serve on soft taco shells with strips of green pepper and onion.

Crockpot Taco Filling

   1 lb. lean ground beef, ground turkey, or ground deer
   1 onion, finely chopped
   2 t. chili powder
   ½ t. oregano
   ½ t. paprika
   ½ t. sea salt
   2 T. allergy-free taco seasoning mix p. 103
   8 oz. tomato sauce

Brown ground meat and drain well. Place in crockpot and add remaining ingredients. Cover and cook 8–12 hours. Serve in taco shells. Top with lettuce, cheese, or cheese alternative and salsa if desired.

Double or triple this recipe, then freeze the leftovers. This will keep frozen for up to 3 months.

Easy Tostadas

10 corn tostadas

16 oz. refried beans

2 c. cooked hamburger or shredded chicken (optional)

1 tomato, diced

1 c. cheese or cheese alternative (optional)

1 c. lettuce, shredded

salsa

sour cream (optional)

Heat refried beans in a small saucepan on medium heat. When warmed, spread beans evenly on tostadas. Top each tortilla with meat, sour cream, salsa, and cheese or cheese alternative. Preheat oven to 400 degrees. Place tostadas on baking sheet or stone. Bake 10–15 minutes, until cheese is melted or chicken is warmed. Serve immediately. Tostadas can be topped with shredded lettuce and fresh diced tomatoes.

I make this when I need a meal in less than 10 minutes. Very quick and easy! Omit the cheese and sour cream for dairy-free tostadas. I vary the ingredients to what I have on hand.

Tacos

    16 oz. refried beans (optional)
     1 lb. cooked hamburger or shredded chicken
     1 tomato, diced
     1 c. lettuce, shredded
     1 c. cheese or cheese alternative (optional)
       salsa
       sour cream (optional)
       avocados (optional)
       corn tortillas
       oil
       diced tomatoes

Fry tortillas in oil until lightly brown on both sides. More oil may be added to the pan as the tortillas cook. Let tortillas dry on a paper towel when done cooking. Layer beans, cheese, lettuce, salsa, and lettuce on tortilla. Enjoy!

Use leftover hamburger or shredded chicken, reheated, to save on time. Use canned beans to save time, although this will cost more. You can use beans or meat that was prepared and frozen ahead of time. For a vegetarian version, omit meat and use refried beans or add cooked black beans.

Black Bean Quesadilla

    3 c. black beans, cooked
    1 c. salsa
    2 c. shredded cheese (optional)
    10 corn tortillas (8 inch)

In a bowl, mash the beans and add salsa. Place 5 tortillas on ungreased baking sheets. Spread the bean mixture on the tortillas. Sprinkle with cheese, if desired, and top with the remaining tortillas. Bake at 350 degrees for 15 to 18 minutes or until crisp and heated through. Cut into wedges. Can be served with sour cream and salsa.

Spaghetti Pizza

    4 c. cooked gluten-free spaghetti (about 1 lb. dry) or rice sticks
    1 egg, lightly beaten
    2 T. milk
    spaghetti sauce

Toppings:

    cheese or cheese alternative
    mushrooms   spinach, chopped
    green peppers   browned hamburger or other cooked meat
    onions   broccoli
    shredded carrots tomatoes

In a bowl, combine pasta, beaten egg and milk. Press into a pie plate and top with spaghetti sauce and desired toppings. Bake for 20 minutes at 350 degrees or until cheese is bubbly.

Great use for leftover pasta!

Chinese Noodles

    8 oz. rice sticks, uncooked
   12 mushrooms, chopped or sliced
    1 T. peanut or other oil
    2 t. minced ginger
    1 T. minced garlic
    1 T. Bragg Liquid Aminos or gluten-free soy sauce (optional)
    1 T. cornstarch
  1 ½ c. chicken broth
  1 ½ c. celery, sliced
  1 ½ c. bean sprouts

Cook and drain rice sticks. Sauté mushrooms, garlic, and minced ginger in a large saucepan or skillet in the peanut oil. In a container with a lid, combine Liquid Aminos, chicken broth, and cornstarch. Shake well. Combine chicken broth mixture with mushrooms and add remaining ingredients. Add rice sticks. Top with 1–2 scallions.

My oldest son refuses to eat spaghetti, but he loves this recipe! The first time I made it, he ate three large helpings and asked for more! This recipe can be used as a side dish or main meal. Cooked beef or chicken can be added to this recipe.

Easy Stir-Fry

    16 oz. package stir-fry vegetable mix, frozen, or fresh vegetables

    2 T. oil

    2 cloves garlic

    3 c. rice, cooked

    Bragg's Liquid Aminos or gluten-free soy sauce

Cook rice as directed. Sauté stir-fry vegetable mix and garlic in oil over medium heat, about 10 minutes. Serve over cooked rice and add about 1 teaspoon Bragg's Liquid Aminos. Serve immediately.

My favorite stir-fry blend contains asparagus, carrots, onions, and green pepper. I could make the same mix by cutting about 1 carrot, 1/2 onion, 1 green pepper, and 1/2 bunch of asparagus, but it is cheaper and takes less time for me to purchase the bag of frozen stir-fry. There are many varieties of frozen stir-fry vegetables available.

Spring Rolls/Egg Rolls

    16 oz. package shredded cabbage (coleslaw mix)*

    8 oz. pork, cooked and drained (optional)

    2 T. oil

    2 cloves of garlic

    ¼ c. onion, finely chopped

    2 T. water

    2 t. cornstarch

    ½ t. sugar

    ¼ t. salt

    1 t. ginger, freshly grated

spring roll wrappers (gluten-free) or egg roll wrappers (not gluten-free)

Heat the oil in a skillet over medium heat. Add the onion and cabbage and sauté for about 10 minutes, until lightly brown. Add garlic and cook, stirring often, for 1 minute. In a separate bowl, combine water, cornstarch, sugar, salt, and ginger. Add to sautéed mixture; cook and stir 1 minute. Add 1/4 cup of mixture to spring roll or egg roll wrappers.

You can also use 2 cups of fresh shredded cabbage plus ½ c. shredded carrot.

Spring Rolls (gluten-free)

Soak spring roll wrappers in water until flexible. Add filling to the center of the spring roll and fold bottom corner over filling, tucking it under on the other side. Fold in the corners over the filling, forming the shape of an envelope. Roll wrapper toward remaining corner. Be sure the wrapper is sealed. Bake spring rolls in the oven at 350 degrees for 20 minutes or until golden brown.

Egg Rolls

Add filling and fold bottom corner over filling, tucking it under on the other side. Fold in the corners over the filling, forming the shape of an envelope. Roll wrapper toward remaining corner. Secure with a small amount of water spread along the edges of the egg roll wrapper. Fry egg rolls in a wok with heated oil until golden brown, approximately 2–3 minutes, turning halfway through.

Fried Rice

3–4 c. cold cooked rice
4 c. eggs, beaten (optional)
3 T. oil, divided
½ c. scallion slices

Other additions to total 1/2 cup:

broccoli	carrots	green beans
sweet potatoes	squash	thawed frozen peas
diced cooked chicken or pork		thawed frozen mixed vegetables

Heat a large skillet over medium heat. Coat the pan with 1 tablespoon oil and heat until very hot. Add eggs. As the edges bubble up, push the outsides to the center, filling the skillet to cook the eggs evenly. Break the cooked eggs into clumps; when set, remove to a bowl. Add 2 tablespoons oil to a hot skillet and heat until hot. Add the rice to the pan, stirring rice to cover it in oil, about 3 minutes. Add cooked eggs, scallions, and 1/2 cup of other ingredients. Serve immediately.

Great for leftover rice, veggies, or eggs. This can be a main dish or a side dish.

Chili Mac

> 1 lb. ground beef
> 1 small onion, chopped
> 15 oz. tomatoes or 2 c. fresh tomatoes, diced
> ½ c. macaroni, uncooked and gluten-free

Brown ground beef and onions until meat is cooked and onions are tender. Stir in tomatoes and macaroni; cover and simmer until macaroni is tender. Salt and pepper to taste.

Quick Chili Mac

> ½ c. cooked gluten free macaroni
> chili

Place cooked macaroni in a bowl. Top with warmed chili. Leftover chili works great for this recipe. Serve immediately. .

My husband introduced me to this combination. His family served chili over pasta. Our southeastern Iowa tradition is to serve peanut butter sandwiches with chili.

Deli Wrap

> 16 slices allergy-free deli meat
> 1 tomato, sliced
> ¼ c. lettuce or spinach, more or less
> 4 tortillas (10 inches)
> 4 T. allergy-free ranch dressing (p. 101) mayonnaise

On a tortilla, spread 1 tablespoon ranch dressing. Place 4 deli meat slices on the dressing. Place tomatoes and lettuce on top of the deli meat. Roll tortilla up tightly to enclose filling. Repeat to make 4 wraps. You may also want to add cheese, cheese alternative, bean sprouts, avocado, shredded carrots, cucumber, or green pepper.

If making ahead of time, wrap individually in plastic wrap and refrigerate. Use approved corn or spelt tortillas if you are gluten-free.

BLT

    1 lb. bacon, gluten-free, without additives or nitrates
    1 tomato, sliced
       lettuce or spinach pieces
       gluten-free bread slices or tortillas
       allergy-free mayonnaise

Cook bacon. Layer on sandwich or tortilla with tomato, lettuce, and mayonnaise. Serve immediately.

Ready-to-Serve Bacon

    1 lb. bacon

Preheat oven to 350 degrees. Place bacon in a single layer on a large baking sheet with rims. Place baking sheet in oven. Cook bacon until brown on both sides. The bacon may need to be turned over halfway through cooking if you are not using a baking stone. Discard grease in a disposable container. Place bacon in a single layer on wax paper (to prevent sticking) and then place the bacon in a freezer-safe container. Freeze until ready to use.

To reheat bacon, microwave 10–15 seconds.

This is a great way to save time! I cook several pounds at a time. It tastes better and isn't as messy as pan-fried bacon. It's perfect for when you need only a slice or two of bacon. This is similar to ready-to-serve bacon found at the grocery store. Great for BLTs!

Corn Dogs

  1 c. gluten-free flour mix
  1 c. corn meal*
  1 t. baking soda
  1 t. salt
  1 t. xanthan gum
  1 egg beaten with ½ c. milk or milk alternative
 12 hotdogs, gluten, additive, and preservative free
    cornstarch**
    oil

Combine gluten-free flour mix, corn meal, baking soda, salt, xanthan gum, egg, and milk or milk alternative until well blended. The batter should not be thin. Add milk if the batter is too thick. Rinse hotdogs and pat dry. Slide a wooden dowel or kabob stick into each hotdog about halfway through the hotdog. Coat the hot dogs with cornstarch. Dip each hotdog into the batter and mold the batter onto the hotdog until the hot dog is coated ¼" thick. Heat approximately ¼ cup of oil in a frying pan or wok to 350 degrees. Place the coated dog immediately into the hot oil. Cook until light golden brown. Turn the corndog, if necessary, until all sides are light golden brown. Drain on paper towels. Serve immediately or freeze corndogs in a freezer-tight bag or container. To reheat frozen corndogs, warm in a 400 degree oven for about 20 minutes.

*Sorghum flour can be substituted for the cornmeal.

**Arrowroot powder, tapioca starch, or potato starch can be substituted for the cornstarch.

To save time, make several extra corndogs and freeze them. When a corndog is needed, simply pull the corndog out of the freezer and bake! The batter for this recipe is somewhat difficult to work with, as it does not stick to the hotdog well before frying, but this gluten-free version of corndogs is well worth the effort.

Sloppy Joes

  1 lb. ground beef, turkey, pork, or deer
  ½ c. onion, finely chopped
  ½ c. green pepper, finely chopped
  8 oz. tomato sauce
  6 oz. tomato paste
  2 T. water
  1 t. chili powder
  ½ t. garlic salt
  1 t. allergy-free Worcestershire sauce (optional)
Dash hot pepper sauce

Brown ground meat; rinse well and drain. Add remaining ingredients and cook in skillet until boiling, then simmer about 5 minutes. Serve on a plate or over buns.

Crockpot method: Place browned and drained ground meat into crockpot. Add ingredients and stir thoroughly. Cover and cook 8–12 hours on low.

This could be made vegetarian by changing the meat to about 2 cups cooked rice.

BBQ Beef Sandwiches

  3 lbs. beef rump roast
  3 T. cornstarch
 15 oz. tomato sauce
  ½ c. finely chopped onions
  ⅓ c. brown sugar, packed
  2 T. lemon juice
  1 T. allergy-free Worcestershire sauce
1 ½ t. chili powder
  1 garlic clove, minced
  1 t. dry mustard.

Rub cornstarch into roast. Place in bottom of crockpot and add remaining ingredients. Cook on low for 14–16 hours. Serve with bread or buns.

Grandma's Italian Beef

    3 lbs. beef roast (do not season)
    2 c. beef broth or water
    1 t. chili powder
    1 t. onion salt
    1 t. garlic salt
    1 t. oregano

Cook roast in oven at 350 degrees, until tender. Cool and slice into thin slices.

Sauce: Mix and simmer the remaining ingredients in a pan on the stove for 5 to 10 minutes. Pour over sliced beef. Bake, covered, at 250 degrees until liquid is cooked down.

Credit is given to my Grandma Levins for this recipe.

Easy Roast

    1 boneless beef or deer roast
    20 oz. chicken or beef broth

Place roast in crockpot. Pour broth over roast. Cook on low for 8 hours. The meat will be very tender. Serve with potatoes or vegetables.

Pot Roast

    1 small potato, sliced
    1 small carrot, sliced
    1 small onion, sliced
      boneless beef roast
      salt and pepper to taste
    2 T. water

Place vegetables in bottom of a crockpot. Salt and pepper the meat and place in the pot. Add water. Cover and cook 10–12 hours.

Coconut Chicken and Rice Bake

> 1 c. water
> ¾ c. cooked brown rice
> ¼ t. paprika
> ¼ t. pepper
> 4 skinless, boneless chicken breasts

1 ½c. canned coconut milk

In a baking dish, mix water, rice, paprika, pepper, and coconut milk.
Place chicken in rice mixture. Sprinkle with additional paprika and
pepper. Bake at 375 degrees for 45 minutes or until rice and chicken are
done. For creamier rice, increase water to 1 1/3 cups.

Chicken Pot Pie

> 2 9" gluten-free pie crusts (if desired)
> 1 c. mixed vegetables, frozen or fresh
> 1 c. diced chicken or turkey
> 1 ¼ c. chicken broth
> ⅓ c. cream soup sauce mix p. 119

Place 1 pie crust in the bottom of a greased 9" pie plate. In a saucepan,
whisk together chicken broth and cream soup sauce ingredients. Bring
to a boil, stirring frequently to prevent sticking. Turn to low and simmer
until thickened. Mix chicken, vegetables, and sauce together;pour into
the pie plate. Top with second pastry sheet and seal the edges. Make slits
at the top of the crust for ventilation. Bake at 350 degrees for 45 minutes
or until crust is golden brown and sauce is bubbly.

*Cream of mushroom soup or a cream soup substitute can be used in place of the
chicken broth and cream soup sauce.*

Crockpot Chicken

  1   carrot, sliced
  1   celery stalk, sliced
  3   thin onion slices
2–3   chicken breasts or thighs
  ½   t. salt
      dash pepper
  2   T. water
      basil leaves

Place vegetables in bottom of crockpot. Arrange chicken pieces on top. Season with salt and pepper. Pour water over all. Sprinkle with basil leaves, if desired. Cover and cook 7–10 hours.

Easy Crockpot Chicken

  1   chicken, frozen

Place unwrapped, frozen chicken in a crockpot. Cover and cook on low heat for 7 to 9 hours. Clean chicken off of the bones and serve the meat.

The raw meat can be frozen for up to 1 year, and the cooked meat can be frozen for up to 3 months. Chop any leftover meat with a food processor or hand chopper and use in chicken salad or slice the meat and use in casseroles, chicken tortilla wraps, or any recipe calling for chicken. Make chicken broth from the leftover liquid and bones in the crock pot.

Chicken Nuggets

 2 c. chicken, cooked and chopped
 1 egg, lightly beaten
 ½ c. gluten-free bread crumbs *
 2 T. olive oil

In a bowl, combine chicken and egg. Roll approximately 2 tablespoons of meat into a ball. Lightly flatten the ball and cover with bread crumbs. Cook in oil on a hot skillet until golden brown, then turn nugget over and brown the other side. Drain on a paper towel until ready to serve.

*Crushed rice crackers, tortilla chips, rice crackers, rice puffs, or rice cereal can be used instead if finely chopped.

Use leftover chicken or turkey to save time in cooking the meat. The chicken can be chopped in the food processor before adding the egg to get a fine texture to the meat. Make extra nuggets and freeze to save time cooking. Nuggets can be frozen for up to 3 months.

Egg Tacos

 8 eggs
 6 corn tortilla shells, fried
 6 allergy-free bacon slices (optional)
 1 c. cheddar cheese or cheese alternative (optional)
   salsa

In a large skillet, scramble or fry eight eggs. When cooked, break the eggs up into small pieces. Add to warmed tortillas. Top with salsa, cheese or cheese alternative, and bacon. Serve immediately.

Cookies, Candy, and Cakes

The majority of the recipes in this section are high in sugar and should be eaten sparingly.

Buckeyes

- ½ c. peanut butter
- 2 c. powdered sugar
- ¾ c. butter, ghee, or allergy-free margarine, separated
- 1 c. allergy-free chocolate chips

Line baking sheet with waxed paper or parchment paper; set aside. In medium bowl, combine peanut butter and 1/2 cup butter until blended. Gradually stir in powdered sugar. On cutting board or flat surface, knead peanut butter mixture until smooth. Shape mixture into 54 (3/4") balls. Arrange balls on prepared baking sheet. Refrigerate 30 minutes. In a small saucepan, melt chocolate and 1/4 cup butter over low heat, stirring occasionally. Using 2 forks, dip balls into chocolate, covering 2/3 of ball and leaving one side exposed to resemble buckeyes. Return to baking sheet. Refrigerate 1 hour or until firm. Store in tightly covered container in refrigerator

Edible Play Dough

- ¾ c. peanut butter or nut butter
- ¾ c. powdered sugar

Mix equal parts peanut butter and powdered sugar until peanut butter is no longer sticky. Use as a play dough or edible snack.

Peanut Butter Play Dough

3 c. powdered sugar

2 c. peanut butter or nut butter

¾ c. honey

In large mixing bowl, combine all ingredients and mix until ingredients are well blended. Turn dough out onto clean work surface; knead like bread dough until play dough is smooth. Store at room temperature in an airtight container. Makes about 4 cups.

Spiced Pecans

½ c. sugar

1 T. ground cinnamon

½ t. salt

1 egg white

1 lb. large pecan halves*

Combine sugar, cinnamon, and salt in a small bowl; set aside. In a large mixing bowl, lightly beat egg white. Add pecans; stir until coated. Sprinkle sugar mixture over pecans; mix well. Spread in a single layer on a baking sheet. Bake at 300 degrees for 20 minutes. Remove nuts while warm to cool on waxed paper. Yield: about 6 cups.

Peanuts can be substituted for the pecans.

Chocolate-Coconut Sauce over Fruit

½ c. coconut milk

½ c. allergy-free chocolate chips

½ t. vanilla extract

1 T. pure maple syrup

1 pint strawberries, washed, stemmed, and quartered

2 ripe bananas, peeled and cut into 3/4" pieces

¼ c. dried unsweetened coconut

Heat the coconut milk in a small saucepan until almost boiling, about 180 degrees. Remove from heat. Add the chocolate chips; cover and let stand for 2 to 3 minutes. Add the vanilla and maple syrup. Whisk until smooth. Divide the strawberries and bananas equally into 4 bowls. Drizzle the chocolate sauce over each serving and sprinkle a tablespoon of the coconut over the top.

The chocolate sauce can also be used as a fruit dip. You may substitute other fruits for the strawberries and bananas.

Bananas on a Stick

ripe bananas

peanut butter or other nut butter

Toppings:

allergy-free mini chocolate chips

sunflower seeds or chopped nuts

shredded coconut

Cut firm, ripe bananas in half and insert a Popsicle stick halfway into each one. Spread peanut butter on at least one side of the banana. Place toppings in individual bowls or plates. Roll each banana in the toppings as desired. Eat immediately.

This is a favorite snack for my children and a favorite snack to make at our Clover Kids 4-H club.

Banana Pops

  4 ripe bananas
  2 T. canola oil
1 ½ c. allergy-free chocolate chips

Toppings:

  sunflower seeds or chopped nuts
  shredded coconut
  sprinkles

Cut 4 firm, ripe bananas in half and insert a Popsicle stick halfway into each one. Set the pops on a wax paper-lined baking sheet and place them in the freezer for 1 hour. In a small saucepan over very low heat, stir together chocolate chips and canola oil until melted. Place toppingsin individual bowls or plates. One at a time, remove the pops from the freezer and, holding them over the saucepan, spoon the chocolate over them. Roll each chocolate-covered banana in a topping, and then return it to the freezer to harden for 1 to 2 hours before serving. Serves 8.

Citrus Berry Sherbet

  2 envelopes unflavored gelatin
  2 c. orange juice
  2 t. lemon juice
  ¼ c. sugar
  2 c. mashed strawberries, fresh or thawed from frozen
  1 c. unsweetened applesauce

Combine orange and lemon juices in a saucepan. Soften gelatin in orange and lemon juice. Add sugar. Stir over low heat until gelatin and sugar are dissolved. Cool. Stir in strawberries and applesauce. Pour into shallow pan. Freeze until firm, about 4 hours. Makes twelve 1/2-cup servings.

Let this freeze completely or it will be like a soft gelatin dessert.

5-Minute Homemade Ice Cream

½ c. kosher salt or coarse sea salt

1 c. milk or milk alternative

2 T. sugar

½ t. vanilla (optional)

   ice cubes

1 small resealable sandwich bag

1 1-gallon resealable freezer bag

Fill the gallon-sized bag half full with ice. Add salt. In the sandwich bag, combine the milk, sugar, and vanilla and seal tightly. Place the sandwich bag inside the gallon-sized bag and seal the large bag so it does not leak. Put on oven mitts or wrap the bag with a dish towel, then shake and roll for about 5 minutes, or until the mixture turns into ice cream. This makes one serving.

You may use more than one sandwich bag inside the gallon-sized bag. This recipe works for most milk types.

If you or your child does not like this ice cream, use the ice cream as a base for a smoothie. In a blender, throw this ice cream, a handful of fruit, , 1 banana, and about 1 cup of juice and blend until smooth. Enjoy!

5-Minute Homemade Sorbet

Follow the same instructions for 5 Minute Ice Cream, but substitute the allergy-free milk with 100% fruit juice, lemonade, or other liquid and, omit the sugar and vanilla.

Raspberry Ice Cream

  2 c. raspberries

  ½ c. milk alternative

1 ½ c. canned coconut milk

  ¼ c. sugar

Combine all ingredients in a blender. Place in freezer-safe container or ice cube tray until frozen. Serve by pureeing in a blender or juicer, or thaw slightly to eat.

Easy Popsicle Treats

100% fruit juice

Popsicle sticks or craft sticks

Container to hold popsicles such as popsicle holders purchased from the store or Dixie™ cups.

Add fruit juice to containers. Place sticks into mixture and freeze until solid. To serve, run container under cold water until the popsicle loosens and falls out. Enjoy!

If you have young children, you may try 1/2 water and 1/2 juice to reduce the sugar content.

Popsicle containers go on sale in midsummer and can be found at most department stores like Wal-Mart or Target. I found a wonderful set on sale at Williams-Sonoma that is made of metal and sturdier than most molds. Dixie cups or small drinking cups can be used, but you have to insert the stick after the popsicle is partially frozen. If you use Dixie cups, simply peel off the paper cup to serve.

Fruit Slush Cups

    1 c. fruit, frozen or fresh

    ½ c. 100% fruit juice, more or less

Place fruit in a freezer-safe container. Cover fruit with fruit juice and freeze overnight. Let thaw several hours before eating.

I created this recipe in high school for my lunches. You can use fresh or frozen fruit and flavored juices. I would freeze them in old yogurt containers and place them in my lunchbox before school. They would be slushy by lunchtime. This recipe works well with mixed fruit.

Easy Fruit Sherbet

    2 c. frozen fruit

    2 T. fruit juice concentrate

Puree frozen fruit and juice concentrate in a food processor or blender until smooth. Add more juice or water if the mix is too thick. Serve immediately or freeze in individual containers for later use.

Many cookie and brownie recipes in this book call for a gluten-free flour mix. Any gluten-free flour mix will work, but Bette Hagman's Featherlight Flour Mix woks best with cookies and cakes. The recipe for her mix is at the beginning of the recipe chapter. For a sweeter taste, use sweet rice flour in place of rice flour in the mix.

Crinkle Cookies

½ c. oil or olive oil

4 squares of unsweetened chocolate

2 c. sugar

4 eggs

2 t. vanilla

2 c. gluten-free flour mix

2 t. baking powder

½ t. salt

1 c. powdered sugar

In a heavy 3-quart saucepan, melt chocolate over low heat until completely melted. Remove from heat. Stir in sugar and coconut oil. Blend in 1 egg at a time until completely blended. Add vanilla, gluten-free flour mix, baking powder, and salt. Mix well. Chill several hours or overnight.

Roll batter into small balls and then roll them in the powdered sugar. Bake 10–12 minutes at 350 degrees.

No-Bake Cookies

½ c. milk or milk alternative

2 c. sugar

3 c. oatmeal*

1 t. vanilla (optional)

½ c. butter, ghee, or allergy-free margarine

⅔ c. peanut butter or other nut butter

6 T. cocoa

Boil milk, sugar, and butter for 1 minute. Mix other ingredients together; stir into boiling mixture quickly. When blended, drop on waxed paper by teaspoon. Let cool, then serve.

Quick-cooking oats are best. Be sure the oats are gluten-free if necessary.

Easy Peanut Butter Cookies

1 c. peanut butter or other nut butter

½ c. honey, sugar, or brown rice syrup

1 egg

1 t. vanilla (optional)

Combine ingredients. Roll into 1/2–1" balls. Place balls on a cookie sheet and press with a fork to flatten. Bake at 350 degrees for 8 to 10 minutes or until lightly brown.

This cookie can be pressed and baked into a large crust for fruit pizzas or tarts.

Pinto Bean Applesauce Raisin Cookies

    1 c. brown sugar

    ½ c. butter, coconut oil, or allergy-free margarine

    2 eggs

    ¾ c. pinto beans, cooked and pureed

    ¾ c. applesauce

2 ¼ c. gluten-free flour mix

    1 t. baking soda

    1 t. baking powder

    ½ t. cinnamon

    ½ c. nuts (optional)

    ½ c. raisins

Cream sugar and butter; add eggs and blend well. Add pureed pinto beans and applesauce; beat until fluffy. Combine dry ingredients in a small bowl; add to creamed mixture and mix until smooth. Stir in nuts and raisins. Drop by tablespoons onto greased cookie sheet. Bake at 375 degrees for 15 to 17 minutes or until golden brown. Cool on rack.

I like to make a large batch of these and freeze most of the cookies. This recipe works great for the "batch and freeze" method. Don't be fooled by the name; kids love these cookies! This recipe is adapted from an internet recipe from the Northharvest Bean Growers Association at www.northharvestbean.org.

Sugar Cookies

1 ½ c. butter, ghee, or coconut oil

2 c. sugar

4 eggs

2 t. vanilla (optional)

2 t. baking powder

1 t. salt

4 t. xanthan gum

5 c. gluten-free flour mix

Mix butter and sugar. Add eggs, vanilla, baking powder, and flour. Scoop dough into balls and bake at 375 degrees for 12 to 14 minutes or until lightly browned. Frost with a buttercream frosting.

This dough can be flattened for cut-out cookies. If the cookie is flattened, it is very crispy and brittle but still tastes wonderful.

Chocolate Chip Quinoa Cookies

¾ c. firmly packed brown sugar

½ c. sugar

1 c. butter, coconut oil, or allergy-free margarine

1 ½ t. vanilla (optional)

1 egg

2 c. gluten-free flour mix

1 t. baking soda

1/2 t. salt

1 c. allergy-free chocolate chips

1/2 c. quinoa, uncooked

Heat oven to 375 degrees. In a large bowl, combine brown sugar, sugar, and butter; beat until light and fluffy. Add vanilla and egg; blend well. Stir in flour, baking soda, and salt; mix well. Stir in chocolate chips and quinoa. Drop dough by teaspoonfuls 2 inches apart onto ungreased cookie sheets. Bake at 375 for 10 to 12 minutes or until light golden brown. Cool 1 minute; remove from cookie sheets.

Oatmeal Chocolate Chip Cookies

   1 c. brown sugar

   1 c. sugar

   ½ c. butter, coconut oil, or allergy-free margarine

   3 eggs

1 ½ c. peanut butter

   1 t. vanilla (optional)

   2 t. baking soda

4 ½ c. oatmeal*

   1 c. allergy-free chocolate chips

In a large mixing bowl, cream together sugar, brown sugar, and butter. Add eggs, vanilla, and peanut butter and blend well. Add baking soda and oatmeal. Stir in chocolate chips. Scoop dough into balls and place on a greased cookie sheet. Bake at 350 degrees 12 minutes or until light golden brown. Remove from the pan gently while still warm. Let the cookies cool.

Quick-cooking oats are best. Be sure the oats are gluten-free if necessary.

Almond-Coconut Sugar Cookies

  1 c. sugar

½ c. coconut oil, butter, or allergy-free margarine

⅓ c. almond milk or other milk alternative

  2 t. vanilla (optional)

¾ c. rice flour

⅓ c. coconut flour

  2 T. tapioca starch or potato starch

½ t. baking powder

½ t. baking soda

½ c. almonds, sliced (optional)

Cream together the coconut oil and sugar. Add vanilla and almond milk. In a separate bowl, combine rice flour, coconut flour, tapioca starch, baking powder, and baking soda. Add dry ingredients to wet ingredients and mix until just blended. Roll into 1" balls and flatten slightly on a greased cookie sheet. Bake 10–12 minutes at 350 degrees. Remove from the pan gently while still warm. Let the cookies cool.

This recipe is based on a recipe found on the back of Bob's Red Mill coconut flour package. Bob's Red Mill is an excellent source of gluten-free flours and baking products.

Gingerbread Cookies

    5 T. butter, ghee, or coconut oil
    ¼ c. brown sugar, packed
    ½ t. cinnamon
    ⅛ t. ground cloves
    1 egg white
    ⅓ c. dark molassas
1 1½ c. gluten-free flour mix
    ½ t. baking soda
    ½ t. baking powder
    ¾ t. salt

Cream butter and sugar. Add egg, spices, salt, and molasses and beat
well. Combine dry ingredients in a separate bowl. Add to butter mixture
and beat well. Preheat oven to 350 degrees. Lightly dust work surface
with rice flour, as the dough will be sticky. Roll the dough to ¼" thick on
top of the rice flour and cut into shapes. Bake for 8 to 10 minutes and
cool on wire racks.

Do not over-bake the cookies.

Fruit Pizza

Crust:

    1 c. peanut butter

    ½ c. honey, sugar, or brown rice syrup

    1 egg

Glaze:

    ½ c. sugar

    ½ t. salt

    2 T. cornstarch

    ½ c. orange juice

    2 T. lemon juice

    ¼ c. water

Filling:

    8 oz. cream cheese

    ½ c. powdered sugar

    2 T. orange juice

Combine ingredients for the crust. Press onto a 9" x 13" cookie sheet. Bake at 350 degrees for 8 to 10 minutes or until lightly brown. Cook glaze until mixture thickens; remove from heat and let cool. Mix together filling ingredients and spread onto crust. Decorate the top with sliced fruit of your choice: grapes, bananas, kiwi, strawberries, mandarin oranges, or other fruit. Spoon glaze over fruit. Keep refrigerated. This recipe contains dairy.

Black Bean Brownies

- ½ c. cocoa powder
- ½ c. butter, coconut oil, or allergy-free margarine
- 2 c. sugar
- 1 c. cooked black beans, pureed
- 4 eggs
- ⅔ c. gluten-free flour mix
- 1 t. salt
- ½ t. baking powder

Mix cocoa, butter, sugar, black bean puree, and eggs together in a bowl until well blended. Sift dry ingredients together; stir into wet mixture. Grease a 9" x 13" pan with cooking spray. Pour the batter into the pan. Bake 350 degrees for 40 minutes or until done. Frost with your favorite chocolate frosting.

I have tried to reduce the sugar in this recipe, but the brownies were not as thick as in the original recipe. This recipe is based on an internet recipe from the Northharvest Bean Growers Association at www.northharvestbean.org.

Brownies

- 3 eggs
- 1 c. sugar
- ½ c. oil (olive or coconut oil works well)
- 2 T. unsweetened cocoa
- ½ c. potato starch
- 1 c. chopped nuts (optional)

Beat eggs and sugar together until light and fluffy. Gradually add oil, then cocoa and potato starch. Stir in chopped nuts. Blend well. Pour mixture into lightly greased 9" square pan. Bake in 350 degree oven for 30 minutes. Cut into squares to serve. The batter will be very thin prior to cooking.

Best-Ever Brownies

    2 eggs

    1 c. coconut oil, butter, or allergy-free margarine

    1 c. white sugar

    1 c. brown sugar

    1 c. gluten-free flour mix

    ⅓ c. cocoa

  1 ½ t. baking powder

  1 ⅓ t. vanilla (optional)

In a saucepan, melt butter or margarine; add cocoa and sugars. Mix well. Add eggs, blending well. Add flour, baking powder, and vanilla. Mix until well blended. Pour into a 9" x 13" pan. Place pecan halves or walnuts on top, if desired. Bake at 350 degrees for 35 to 40 minutes.

Peanut Butter Brownies

    1 c. peanut butter

    ½ c. honey, sugar, or brown rice syrup

    1 t. baking soda

    2 eggs

    1 t. vanilla (optional)

Combine ingredients and pour into a 9" pan. Bake at 350 degrees for 20 to 25 minutes. Top with peanut butter frosting p. 194.

Pumpkin Peanut Butter Bars

    1 c. peanut butter

    ½ c. honey, sugar, or brown rice syrup

    1 t. baking soda

    2 eggs

    1 t. vanilla (optional)

    ½ c. pumpkin or squash, cooked and mashed

Combine ingredients and pour into a 9" pan. Bake at 350 degrees for 20 to 30 minutes. Top with peanut butter frosting p. 194.

Chocolate Peppermint Sticks

  2 squares unsweetened chocolate *

  ½ c butter, coconut oil, or allergy-free margarine

  2 eggs, beaten

  1 c. sugar

  ¼ t. peppermint flavoring or Grade-A peppermint essential oil**

dash salt

  ½ c. ground almonds (optional)

  ½ c. gluten-free flour mix

Melt chocolate and butter or margarine together. Add remaining ingredients. Bake in a greased 9" pan for 20 to 25 minutes at 350 degrees. Cool completely. Spread icing over the top.

Icing:

  2 T. butter, ghee, or allergy-free margarine

  1 c. powdered sugar

  ¼ t. peppermint flavoring or Grade-A peppermint essential oil

  1 T. allergy-free milk

Put in refrigerator to set. When the icing is set, drizzle over the top 1 square of chocolate and 1 tablespoon of butter, ghee, or allergy-free margarine melted together. Refrigerate.

*Unsweetened chocolate can be substituted with 6 teaspoons cocoa blended with 2 tablespoons butter or margarine.

**Peppermint essential oil can only be used if the oil is labeled "food grade." Do not use low-quality oils. I use oils from Young Living Essential Oils.

I adapted this recipe from my great-grandmother's original, which was used frequently in her catering business. It looks complicated but is very easy to make, and the gluten-free, dairy-free version is well liked by all. This recipe can be frozen.

Peanut Butter Crunch Bars

  3 ¼ c. powdered sugar

   ½ c. butter or allergy-free margarine

  16 oz. peanut butter or other nut butter

   3 c. crispy cereal or corn flakes

  16 oz. allergy-free chocolate chips (optional)

Melt butter over low heat in saucepan. In a mixing bow, blend peanut butter and sugar. Add the melted butter and continue to blend. Stir in cereal. Spread mixture evenly onto a 9" x 13" pan. In a separate saucepan, melt the chocolate chips over low heat. Spread melted chocolate evenly over bars. Refrigerate to cool. Cut into bars. Makes approximately 30 bars.

I got this recipe from the cap of Smucker's Natural Peanut Butter jar. It is very good. I have made it with both peanut and other nut butters, and it works well either way. This recipe is high in sugar.

Sylvia's Rhubarb Torte

   1 c. gluten-free flour mix

   ½ c. butter, coconut oil, or allergy-free margarine

   3 T. powdered sugar

      pinch of salt

Mix all ingredients with handheld mixer until crumbly. Bake in an 8" x 8" pan for 10 minutes at 375 degrees. While the crust is in the oven, beat together the following:

   2 eggs

 1 ½ c. sugar

   ¼ c. gluten-free flour mix

   ¾ t. baking powder

Take the crust out of the oven and add 3 cups of sliced rhubarb on top. Pour the egg, sugar, and flour mixture on top of the rhubarb and bake 30–40 minutes at 375 degrees.

This recipe is adapted from a recipe given to me by Sylvia Graber.

Pear Cranberry Crisp

  3 pears, peeled, cored, and cut into chunks
  1 c. whole cranberries
  ¼ c. maple syrup
  2 T. lemon juice
  ½ c. oatmeal (gluten-free)*
  ¼ c. brown sugar
  1 T. flour
  1 T. butter, ghee, or allergy-free margarine

Preheat oven to 400 degrees. In a medium bowl, combine the pears, cranberries, maple syrup, and lemon juice; toss. Set aside. In another bowl, combine the oatmeal, brown sugar, and flour. Cut in the butter until the consistency resembles coarse crumbs and the dough just barely holds together. Spoon the cranberry mixture into an 8" x 8" baking dish; spoon the dry mixture over it. Bake for 10 minutes or until the topping is brown and crisp. Reduce the heat to 350 degrees and bake for 20 to 25 minutes more or until fruit is bubbly.

*An allergy-free cereal (crushed) can be used in place of the oatmeal, if desired. Cereals such as Rice Crunch Ems, Rice Twice, corn flakes will all work well for this.

Coconut Vanilla Donuts

- ¾ c. rice flour
- ¼ c. garbanzo bean flour
- ¼ c. potato starch
- ¼ c. arrowroot powder
- 1 ½ t. baking powder
- ¼ t. baking soda
- ½ t. zanthan gum
- ¼ t. salt
- ½ c. So Delicious® Dairy Free Vanilla Coconut Milk
- 1 c. organic raw cane sugar
- ⅓ cup coconut oil + extra for greasing
- ½ cup unsweetened applesauce or pear sauce
- 1 t. vanilla extract (optional)
- ½ c. unsweetened coconut flakes.

Grease a donut pan with coconut oil and preheat oven to 350 degrees. Combine the first 8 ingredients in a bowl. In a medium pot, add milk and coconut oil and warm over low heat until the coconut oil melts. Do not allow this to boil. Mix gently with a wooden spoon while warming. Once the oil is melted, remove from heat and add in the sugar. Stir together until sugar is dissolved completely. Add applesauce and vanilla extract and stir to combine. Pour the liquid mixture into the dry ingredients and mix gently until combined together well. (An emersion blender can be used to make the batter smooth if clumps form in the batter.) Add coconut flakes and mix with a wooden spoon. Pour into a greased donut pan and fill about half way. Bake for 15 minutes at 350 degrees. Allow to cool for 15 to 30 minutes before removing from the pan.

Glaze: and ½ cup powdered sugar into a small bowl and add 1-2 T. of hot water. Mix well to combine. Coat the donuts thinly with the glaze. The donuts can be sprinkled with coconut flakes, if desired.

Make extra doughnuts and freeze them. They can be thawed and eaten or heated and served warm. If you don't have a donut pan, you can use a cupcake pan to bake them in. This recipe is based from the recipe book So Delightful by So Delicious® Dairy Free.

Buttercream Frosting

    4 ½ c. powdered sugar

    6 T. butter, ghee, or allergy-free margarine at room temperature

    1 ½ t. vanilla (optional)

    ¼ c. milk or milk alternative

Beat butter until light and fluffy. Gradually add half the powdered sugar, beating well. Beat in the milk and vanilla. Gradually beat in remaining sugar, adding milk if needed. This will frost a 9" x 13" cake, a two-layer 9" cake, or 24 cupcakes.

Variation: For chocolate buttercream frosting, add 2 ounces of melted, cooled unsweetened chocolate along with the vanilla.

Fluffy Buttercream Frosting

    1 ½ c. powdered sugar

    ¼ c. butter, ghee, or allergy-free margarine at room temperature

    ¼ c. Spectrum shortening or other non-hydrogenated shortening (Do not use Crisco™)

    2 T. milk or milk alternative

Beat butter and shortening until fluffy. Add sugar and beat 3 minutes. Add vanilla and milk; beat 5 minutes.

Peanut Butter Frosting

    1 ¼ c. powdered sugar

    3 T. peanut butter or other nut butter

    1 t. vanilla (optional)

    2 T. milk or milk alternative

Beat all ingredients in a mixing bowl until well blended and smooth. If the mixture is too thick, add more milk. If it is too thin, add more powdered sugar.

Tara's Gluten-Free Pie Crust

¾ c. tapioca flour

¾ c. cornstarch

1 c. rice flour

1 t. salt

1 t. sugar (omit if making a savory dish)

1 c. butter or allergy-free margarine

¼–½ c. ice water

Combine dry ingredients in a food processor. Add butter; grind 8–10 seconds. Add ice water until dough holds tighter. Refrigerate at least 1 hour.

This mix can be combined by hand, but it is easier with a food processor. If the dough is too sticky, lay the dough between two sheets of plastic wrap then roll the dough out. You can also dust the dough with rice flour to make it less sticky.

Cookie Pie Crust

2 T. sugar

½ c. butter, coconut oil, or allergy-free margarine, melted

1½ c. gluten-free cookies, finely crushed

Combine all the ingredients. Blend well. Press into bottom of an ungreased 9" round pan. Add pie filling and bake or freeze the crust until ready to use.

Shortbread Pie Crust

3 T. sugar

2 T. milk or milk alternative

½ c. butter, coconut oil, or allergy-free margarine, melted

1½ c. gluten-free cookies, finely crushed

Combine all the ingredients. Blend well. Press into bottom of an ungreased 9" round pie pan. Add pie filling and bake or freeze the crust until ready to use.

Pumpkin Pie

¼ c. sugar

1 t. ground cinnamon

½ t. salt

½ t. ground ginger

¼ t. ground cloves

2 eggs

1 (15 oz.) can or 2 c. pumpkin puree

1 c. canned coconut milk *

Mix sugar, cinnamon, salt, ginger, and cloves in a small bowl. Beat eggs in a large bowl. Stir in pumpkin and sugar-spice mixture. Combine canned coconut milk. Pour into (2) 9" pie crusts. Bake in a preheated 425-degree oven for 15 minutes. Reduce temperature to 350 degrees and bake 40–50 minutes or until knife inserted near center comes out clean. Cool. Serve immediately or refrigerate. Makes 8 servings.

Make this pie ahead of time and freeze until ready to use. Reheat by thawing overnight in a refrigerator and then bake until the pie is heated through, about 20 minutes.

*For a substitute, combine 1 cup of milk alternative powder (such as DariFree) and 3/4 cup hot water in a blender or mix 1 cup powdered milk and ½ cup water.

Strawberry Pie

   1 ½ c. water
   1 c. sugar
   2 T. cornstarch
   1 T. grape juice concentrate
   3 T. gelatin
   4 c. strawberries, whole or sliced
      baked pie crust

Bring water, sugar, cornstarch, and grape juice to a boil in a saucepan. Remove from heat and add gelatin. Put strawberries in pie crust. Pour mixture over strawberries. Refrigerate.

Apple Crisp or Apple Pie

   5 c. apples, peeled and sliced
   ½ c. sugar
   ½ t. cinnamon
   ⅛ t. nutmeg

   Topping:
   ¼ c. sugar
   ¼ c. gluten-free flour mix
   ⅛ c. butter, ghee, or allergy-free margarine, softened

Mix apples, sugar, cinnamon, and nutmeg together. If using a pie shell, pour mixture into the shell; otherwise, pour mixture into an 8" x 8" greased baking pan. In a separate bowl, mix sugar and flour. Cut butter into the sugar and flour mixture until the mixture resembles coarse crumbs; sprinkle on top of apple mixture. Bake at 400 degrees for 40 minutes.

Pie Crust Treats

    uncooked piecrust

    jam

Tear pie crust into 2" pieces and press into the bottom of a mini muffin tin. If you are using a gluten-free crust, you may need to "plop" it into the muffin tin and spread in a thin layer. Place about 1 tablespoon of jam in the center of the crust. Bake at 350 degrees for 20 minutes or until the crust is browned and the jam is bubbly.

Almond Cookie Tart Crust

    1 c. ground almonds

    1 c. gluten-free flour mix

    ½ c. granulated sugar

    ½ c. butter, coconut oil, or allergy-free margarine

    1 egg yolk, lightly beaten

    ½ t. vanilla

Grease a pie pan. In a food processor, combine almonds, flour, and sugar. Add butter and pulse until mixture resembles coarse texture. Pour egg yolks and vanilla over and combine just until mixture can be formed by hand into a mass. Press mixture into bottom and up the sides of the pan. Crust will be about 1/4" thick. Preheat oven to 350 degrees and bake 10–12 minutes. Will be lightly browned around edges and just partially baked. If using immediately, add toppings and finish baking or refrigerate or freeze until needed. Peach tart topping (below) can be used with this recipe.

Peach Tart Topping

   3 T. peach preserves, jam, or jelly, divided
   ¼ c. sliced almonds
4–5 large peaches, skinned and sliced
   3 T. sugar (less if peaches are sweet)
   2 T. butter, ghee, or allergy-free margarine

Spread 2 tablespoons of peach preserves over cooled almond cookie tart crust. Arrange peach slices, overlapping or stacked over preserves. Heat 1 tablespoon of preserves and brush over peaches. Sprinkle with sugar and sliced almonds. Dot peaches with bits of butter over the top. Bake in 350-degree oven for 20 minutes or until peaches are just tender. Serve warm, at room temperature, or chilled.

This recipe can be used as a topping for almond cookie tart crust, as a pie filling, or in fruit cobbler.

Fruit Cobbler

- ¾ c. white rice flour
- ¼ c. potato starch or tapioca starch
- ½ t. xanthan gum
- ½ t. salt
- 1 t. baking powder
- ⅔ c. butter, ghee or allergy-free margarine
- 1 T. sugar
- ¾ c. water
- 1 egg
- your favorite pie filling

Preheat oven to 425 degrees. Generously grease a 10" pie pan; set aside. Place all ingredients in a small mixing bowl. Beat 2 minutes on medium speed. Spread batter in prepared pie pan. Carefully spoon pie filling into center of batter. Do not stir. Bake for 35 minutes, until crust is golden brown.

If you do not have pie filling, simply use 3–4 cups of fruit, 1 tablespoon lemon juice, and 1/2–1 cup of sugar combined and brought to a boil in a saucepan. Use this as the filling.

In a Jar Mixes

Yellow Cake in a Jar

In a pint jar, combine the following:

1 ¼ c. gluten-free flour mix (rice or sweet rice mix is best)

2 t. baking powder

½ t. baking soda

½ t. xanthan gum

½ t. salt

⅔ c. sugar

Place jar in dark, dry area until ready to use.

When ready to use, add:

2 eggs

1 c. mayonnaise

In a bowl, beat eggs until light and fluffy. Add mayonnaise and mix until well blended. Add pint jar mix and blend just until combined. Do not over-mix. Pour into a greased 8" pan. Bake at 350 degrees for 30 to 35 minutes.

This is a great cake recipe! Usually, I mix one to use and mix 1–3 more into jars for future use. Perfect for traveling or if you are in a hurry. Make several jars of this recipe at the same time and store until ready to use.

Chocolate Cake in a Jar

In a pint jar, combine the following:

- 1½ c. gluten-free flour mix (rice or sweet rice mix is best)
- ⅓ c. unsweetened cocoa
- ¼ t. baking powder
- ½ t. baking soda
- 1 t. xanthan gum
- ⅞ c. sugar

Place jar in dark, dry area until ready to use.

When ready to use, add:

- 1 egg
- ½ c. mayonnaise
- ½ t. vanilla
- 5 oz. water

In a bowl, beat eggs until light and fluffy. Add mayonnaise and mix until well blended. Add vanilla. Alternately add pint jar mix and water, blending just until combined. Do not over-mix. Pour into a greased 8" pan or in muffin pan. Bake cake at 350 degrees for 25 to 30 minutes. Bake cupcakes for 15 to 20 minutes.

Sugar Cookies in a Jar

In a pint jar, combine the following:

- ½ c. sugar
- ½ t. baking powder
- ¼ t. salt
- 1 t. xanthan gum
- 1 ¼ c. gluten-free flour mix

Place jar in dark, dry area until ready to use.

When ready to use, add:

- 6 T. butter or allergy-free margarine at room temperature
- 1 egg
- ½ t. vanilla (optional)

In a bowl, beat butter or margarine until light and fluffy. Add egg and vanilla. Add pint jar mix and blend just until combined. Do not over-mix. Scoop dough into balls and bake at 375 degrees for 12 to 14 minutes or until lightly browned. Frost with a buttercream frosting.

This dough can be flattened for cutout cookies. If the cookie is flattened, it is very crispy and brittle but still tastes wonderful.

Almond Coconut Sugar Cookies in a Jar

In a pint jar, combine the following:

2 c. sugar

¾ c. rice flour

⅓ c. coconut flour

2 T. potato or tapioca starch

½ t. baking powder

½ t. baking soda

Place jar in dark, dry area until ready to use.

When ready to use, add:

½ c. coconut oil, butter, or allergy-free margarine

⅓ c. almond milk or other milk alternative

t. vanilla (optional)

½ c. almonds, sliced (optional)

In a bowl, beat coconut oil, butter, or margarine until light and fluffy. Add vanilla. Alternately add pint jar mix and milk or milk alternative; blend just until combined. Add sliced almonds if desired. Do not over-mix. Roll into 1" balls and flatten slightly on a greased cookie sheet. Bake 10–12 minutes at 350 degrees. Remove from the pan gently while still warm. Let the cookies cool.

Gluten-Free Bread for Machine in a Bag

Combine the following dry ingredients in a container or plastic bag that seals. There are approximately 2 cups of flour per pound, so 25 pounds of flour will yield approximately 15 batches. Add the specified amount to each container or bag and store in a cool dry place until ready to use.

3 ⅛ c. gluten-free flour mix
1 ½ t. salt
3 ½ t. xanthan gum
2 T. brown sugar
¼ t. ascorbic acid (optional)

When ready to make bread, have these ingredients:

3 eggs, beaten
1 ⅛ c. warm water
3 T. oil
2 ¼ t. or 1 packet yeast

When ready to make bread, combine the water and yeast first. Combine the eggs and oil and then add the water and yeast mixture. Next, add the dry mix that was stored in the container or bag.

Place ingredients in bread machine according to manufacturer's directions. Press start button.

Classic Pancakes in a Jar

In a pint jar, combine the following:

- ¾ c. gluten-free flour mix
- 2 t. baking powder
- ¼ t. xanthan gum
- ¼ t. salt
- 1 t. sugar

When ready to make pancakes, measure out ¾ cup plus 4 teaspoons of dry mix into a bowl. Then add:

- 2 eggs, well beaten
- ½ c. milk alternative
- 2 T. oil

Beat together eggs, milk, and oil. Add this mixture to the dry mix that has been measured out; stir until all ingredients are well blended. Cook on hot griddle. Be sure to spread the batter to make it thin on the griddle, or the middle may not get cooked evenly.

Around the House

Gluten-Free Paper-Mache Glue #1

 1 T. cornstarch

 1 liter water, boiled

 1 t. cold water

Boil one liter of water. Put the cornstarch into the mixing bowl and, while mixing, gradually add a small amount of cold water until the cornstarch becomes a smooth, creamy paste. While mixing, gradually pour the boiling water into the cornstarch paste. You can start using the glue when it is cool enough to touch.

Gluten-Free Paper-Mache Glue #2

 1 c. Elmer's Glue or other gluten-free glue

 ½ c. water

Combine the glue and water. To use: tear sheets of newspaper into strips and dip them into the glue. It is easier to tear newspaper into neat strips when you tear along the grain of the paper. Try tearing the newspaper both vertically and horizontally to discover which way the grain runs. Attach the strip of newspaper to the object you would like to paper-mache. We use a balloon that is blown up. Attach the paper to the balloon. When the paper dries, cut a hole in the top of the paper-mache and be sure to pop the balloon. Fill the paper-mache shell with candy, stickers, or prizes, and you have a piñata.

Gluten-Free Play Dough

- ½ c. rice flour
- ½ c. cornstarch
- ½ c. salt
- 2 t. cream of tartar
- 1 c. water
- 1 t. cooking oil

Mix ingredients. Cook and stir on low heat for 3 minutes or until it forms a ball. Cool completely before storing in a sealable plastic bag or well-sealed container.

This play dough works well and has a long storage life. Great for school!

Laundry Detergent

- 6 c. water
- ⅓ bar of Ivory soap, grated
- ½ c. washing soda
- ½ c. borax
- 4 c. hot water
- 22 c. (5 quarts + 2 c.) hot water, separated
- 2 gallon bucket

Mix Ivory soap in a saucepan with 6 cups water and heat on low until dissolved. Stir in washing soda and borax. Stir until thickened; remove from heat. Add 4 cups hot water to the 2-gallon bucket. Add soap mixture and mix well. Fill bucket with hot water and mix well. Set aside for 24 hours or until mixture thickens. Use ½ cup of mixture per load.

This laundry detergent works well in cleaning clothes but does not work well for heavily soiled or stained items. It is very inexpensive to make. I have been using this recipe for many years.

Bibliography

Arthur, Michael, Kathy Gaskin, Lew Kidder and Jean Marvel, eds. *Uprisings: the Whole Grain Bakers' Book.* New York, NY: Bantam, 1983. Print.

Ball Blue Book of Preserving. Muncie, IN: Alltrista Consumer Products, 2003. Print.

"Celiac Disease | American Celiac Disease Alliance." **Welcome | American Celiac Disease Alliance**. Web. Spring 2009. <http://americanceliac.org/celiac-disease/>.

"Cookbook:Vegan Substitutions - Wikibooks, Open Books for an Open World." *Wikipedia, the Free Encyclopedia.* Web. 18 Nov. 2010. <http://en.wikipedia.org/wiki/B:Cookbook:Vegan_Substitutions>.

"Egg Allergy." *KidsHealth - the Web's Most Visited Site about Children's Health.* Web. Spring 2010. <http://kidshealth.org/teen/food_fitness/nutrition/egg_allergy.html>.

"Egg Allergy." *KidsHealth - the Web's Most Visited Site about Children's Health.* Web. Spring 2010. <http://kidshealth.org/kid/nutrition/diets/egg_allergy.html>.

Emily. "Coconut Drink Recipe | Joyful Abode." Blog | *Joyful Abode.* Web. 20 Jan. 2011. <http://www.joyfulabode.com/2009/10/11/coconut-drink-recipe/>.

"Food Allergy or Food Intolerance?" *National Institute of Allergy and Infectious Diseases Home Page.* Web. 06 May 2008. <http:// www.niaid.nih.gov/topics/foodAllergy/understanding/Pages/foodIntolerance.aspx>.

Frandsen, Betty Rae., Kathryn J. Frandsen, and Kent P. Frandsen. *Where's Mom Now That I Need Her?: Surviving Away from Home.* Sandy, UT: Aspen West Pub. & Distribution, 1983. Print.

"Grains and Flours Glossary." *Celiac Sprue Association.* Web. 25 Feb. 2011. <http://www.csaceliacs.org/gluten_grains.php>.

Hagman, Bette. *The Gluten-free Gourmet Cooks Fast and Healthy: Wheat-free Recipes with Less Fuss and Fat.* New York: Henry Holt, 2000. Print

Hagman, Bette. *The Gluten-free Gourmet Bakes Bread: More than 200 Wheat-free Recipes.* New York: Henry Holt, 1999. Print.

"Living Without - Substitutions." *Living Without - Gluten-Free, Dairy-Free and Other Food Allergies.* Web. 20 Jan. 2011. <http://www.livingwithout.com/resources/substitutions.html>.

Mayo Clinic Staff "Food Intolerance or Food Allergy?" 4 Dec. 2007 Mayo Clinic. http://www.mayoclinic.org/news2007-mchi/4367.html

Pinto Bean Applesauce Raisin Cookies. US Dry Bean Council, n.d. Web. Fall 2006. <http://www.usdrybeans.com/2010/08/pinto-bean-applesauce-raisin-cookies/>.

Prideaux, Lucy-Ann. "Food Intolerance" EzineArticles.com 20 July 2005 http://ezinearticles.com/?Food-Intolerance&id=52605

"Wheat Free and Gluten Free Flours." *Wheat-free.org - Wheat Free Recipes, Places to Eat, Suppliers of Ingredients.* Web. 25 Feb. 2011. <http://www.wheat-free.org/wheat-free-flour.html>.

Yaron, Ruth. *Super Baby Food: Absolutely Everything You Should Know about Your Baby and Toddler from Starting Solid Foods to Age Three Years.* Peckville, PA: F. J. Roberts Pub., 2002. Print.

A

Alternatives

Appetizers and Snacks

Around the House

Breads and Baked Goods

Cookies, Candy, and Cakes

Condiments

Fruits and Vegetables

Salad

House Salad, 114
Italian Pasta Salad, 113
Mock Jell-O™, 116

Soups
Chicken Soup, 120
Dairy-Free Cream Soup Substitute #1, 119
Dairy-Free Cream Soup Substitute #2 (Single Serving), 119
Dairy-Free Cream Soup Substitute #3 (Single Serving), 120
Kevin's Chili, 122
Old-Fashioned Bean Soup, 120
Red Pepper Soup, 122
Tortilla Soup, 121
Vegetable Beef Soup, 123
Vegetable Slaw with Apricot Dressing, 114
Vegetarian Chili, 121